ARTHROGRAPHY OF THE SHOULDER

ARTHROGRAPHY OF

THE SHOULDER

*The Diagnosis and
Management of the
Lesions Visualized*

By

JULIUS S. NEVIASER, M.D.

*Clinical Professor of Orthopaedic Surgery,
George Washington University Medical School*

*Formerly Consultant-Lecturer at the U. S.
Naval Hospital, Bethesda, Maryland and the
Walter Reed Army Hospital, Washington, D. C.*

*Past Chairman of the Department of Orthopaedic
Surgery at the Washington Hospital Center,
Washington, D. C. and the Prince George's
General Hospital, Cheverly, Maryland*

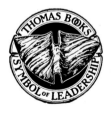

CHARLES C THOMAS • PUBLISHER
Springfield • Illinois • U.S.A.

Published and Distributed Throughout the World by

CHARLES C THOMAS · PUBLISHER

Bannerstone House

301-327 East Lawrence Avenue, Springfield, Illinois, U.S.A.

© *1975, by* CHARLES C THOMAS · PUBLISHER

ISBN 0-398-03304-8

Library of Congress Catalog Card Number: 74-12117

*With THOMAS BOOKS careful attention is given to all details of manufacturing
and design. It is the Publisher's desire to present books that are satisfactory as to
their physical qualities and artistic possibilities and appropriate for their particular
use. THOMAS BOOKS will be true to those laws of quality that assure a good
name and good will.*

Printed in the United States of America

K-8

Library of Congress Cataloging in Publication Data

Neviaser, Julius S.
    Arthrography of the shoulder.

    Bibliography: p.
    1. Shoulder joint—Diseases. 2. Joints—Radiography.
I. Title. [DNLM: 1. Shoulder joint—Radiography.
WE810 N521a]
RC932.N48   616.7'2   74-12117
ISBN 0-398-03304-8

Dedicated to my wife, Jane, the mother of our three sons, Jules, Robert and Thomas, all orthopaedic surgeons. Her patience and understanding are infinite.

PREFACE

THIS BOOK REPRESENTS the culmination of my lifelong interest in the shoulder joint. When I was a resident, the terms "Frozen Shoulder" or "Periarthritis of the Shoulder" were meaningless. None of my teachers could explain the pathologic anatomy of this condition. After a thorough study of a series of cases in the operating room as well as at the autopsy table, I published the results of the pathological findings in 1945. At that time it was suggested that the term "Adhesive Capsulitis" would be more descriptive of the lesion than that of "Frozen Shoulder." Further study of various conditions of the shoulder joint convinced me that arthrography was the one procedure which would help in establishing a definite diagnosis in the many instances where such terms as bursitis, neuritis and arthritis were used indiscriminately.

I am grateful to the members of the Department of Radiology of the Washington Hospital Center and the former Emergency Hospital for their generous cooperation. It was at these two institutions that most of this work was done. I wish to express my gratitude to Mr. Victor Landi, who over the years has made most of the photographs and illustrations for my articles as well as for this book.

My son, Robert, reviewed the manuscript and made many helpful suggestions. As a father to a son I can only say thank you. Some of my colleagues who referred many interesting cases to me deserve my sincere appreciation. All credit and deserving acknowledgement is due my office staff for their meticulous attention in maintaining accurate records of the many cases seen and the typing and retyping of the manuscript.

Finally, to the Publishers, especially Mr. Payne Thomas, for their encouragement and helpful thoughts in the preparation of this book.

JULIUS S. NEVIASER

INTRODUCTION

THE PURPOSE of this manuscript is to emphasize to the reader the value of arthrography of the shoulder joint. It is my belief that arthrography of the shoulder offers more real clinical information to the orthopaedic surgeon or to the radiologist than performing this procedure on any other joint. Yet, despite the value of this relatively simple study, it is not being used as often as it should. Its infrequent use could stem from the fact that the technique may not be familiar to many who wish to use it or from the lack of expertise in the interpretation of the arthrograms. I have seen the latter point well illustrated in the Department of Radiology of the hospital where I do most of my arthrographies. In many instances I have disagreed with the radiologists in their readings of the films and my interpretations have been proven correct at the operating table. This volume is written to encourage the use of arthrography and to pass on to the reader the lessons learned from my personal experience in performing over three thousand arthrographies and the knowledge of the anatomy of the shoulder gained at postmortem examination and in the operating room.

Arthrography of the shoulder is not a new procedure. Codman (1934) in his great masterpiece, "The Shoulder," mentions the possibility of injecting an opaque fluid into the shoulder joint to confirm the diagnosis of a rupture of the supraspinatus tendon. Although he did not try this procedure, he indicated, on the cover design of his book, the appearance of the joint in cases of complete tear. Many European surgeons such as Lindblom and Palmer, Oberholzer, Axen, Frostad and Pettersson have published various articles on this subject, outlining their different techniques and roentgenographic findings. Oberholzer used arthrograms of the shoulder in order to study the lesions caused by a dislocation or subluxation. Lindblom and Palmer used arthrography as a method of detecting complete or incomplete ruptures in the tendinous aponeurosis of the shoulder joint and in the tendon of the long head of the biceps. Axen reported his use of arthrography and stressed the value of his technique in diagnosing ruptures of the capsular ligament of the joint and the tendon of the long head of the biceps on the basis of the material found in 173 cases. He stated that a communication between the subdeltoid bursa and joint may be present in individuals advanced in years without evidence of trauma or clinical symptoms. Incidentally, this is now common knowledge to those surgeons interested in the shoulder. In this article, however, the illustrations were sparse and of poor quality. This was a common finding with most of the previous authors. Pettersson, in an excellent monograph on the rupture of the tendinous aponeurosis in anterior-inferior dislocations of the shoulder, used arthrography quite frequently to test for cuff ruptures, particularly if the patients were over thirty years of age. He also used it to demonstrate the progress of healing in the torn capsule at the anterior-inferior part of the joint.

Kernwein presented a paper on arthrographic studies of the shoulder joint before the American Orthopaedic Association in Banff, Alberta, Canada in June, 1956, in which he outlined the results of the studies he and his associates made on ninety-six problem shoulders. I had the opportunity to discuss this paper and emphasized the value of the axillary view in this procedure. I believe this article, subsequently published in the *Journal of Bone and Joint Surgery,* gave added impetus to the use of arthrography as a tool in the diagnosis of some shoulder lesions.

CONTENTS

ARTHROGRAPHY OF THE SHOULDER

Chapter One

ANATOMY

A KNOWLEDGE OF THE ANATOMY of the shoulder joint will not only help the surgeon or radiologist in the technique of arthrography but will be invaluable in interpreting the arthrograms. The stability of the shoulder is maintained primarily by soft tissue structures. The most important structure is the articular capsule which completely envelops the shoulder joint. It is remarkably loose and this accounts for much of the free movement of the joint in all directions. The capsule is prolonged downward in the form of a fold in the dependent position of the arm (Fig. 1). When the arm is abducted, this fold becomes obliterated and the capsule becomes tense (Fig. 2). The capsule is closely adherent to the neck of the glenoid anteriorly where it blends with the glenoid labrum, which is a reinforcement of the capsule about the glenoid rim, and joins the periosteum about the scapular neck. It does however, have some redundancy near the neck of the scapula posteriorly as seen in Figure 8. I have often speculated that this anatomical feature may be a reason why there is less frequency of posterior dislocation of the shoulder. Since there is more room to displace the humeral head posteriorly, stretching or tearing of the posterior portion of the capsule is less likely to occur.

The synovial membrane lines the fibrous layer of the capsule. It extends from the margins of the glenoid cavity over the inner surface of the capsule and covers the lower part and sides of the anatomical neck of the humerus, where it is reflected toward the margins of the articular cartilage of the humeral head. The synovial sheath of the long head of the biceps tendon is an extension of the joint capsule and the subscapularis bursa is an outpouching of the capsule (Fig. 3). Thus, any pathologic process of the synovial lining of the capsule could involve the bursa or biceps sheath or both. On all aspects, except the inferior, the capsular ligament,

3

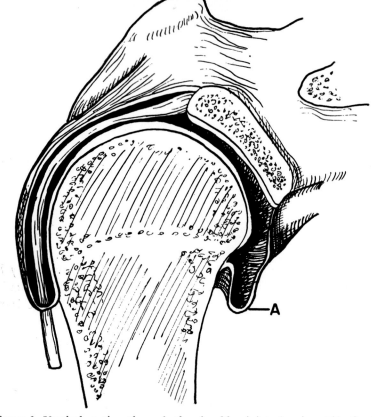

Figure 1. Vertical section through the shoulder joint showing (A) the fold of the capsule of the joint with synovial membrane lining its inner surface. (Courtesy of *J Bone Joint Surgery, 27*:211, 1945.)

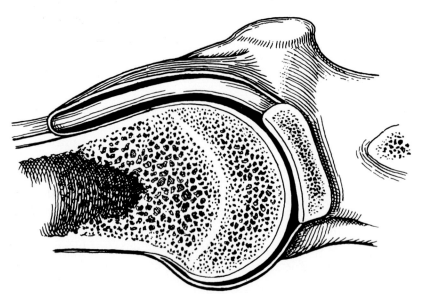

Figure 2. A vertical section through the shoulder joint showing obliteration of the dependent fold with the arm in abduction. (Courtesy of *A.A.O.S. Instructional Course Lectures, 6*:281, 1949.)

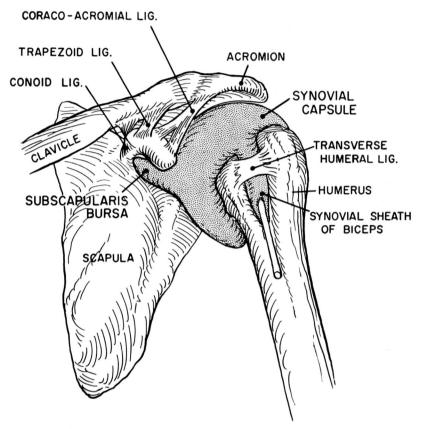

Figure 3. The synovial capsule about the shoulder joint reveals its outpouching as the subscapularis bursa as well as its prolongation to form the sheath of the biceps tendon.

which includes the three glenohumeral ligaments, is supported by muscles, the tendons of which are intimately connected with it. This intimate union of the tendons of the external rotators, the supraspinatus, infraspinatus and teres minor, with the internal rotator, the subscapularis, converts them into supporting ligaments of the shoulder. This entire enveloping structure is called the musculotendinous cuff or rotator cuff of the shoulder.

The only landmarks one needs to be familiar with in performing arthrographies are the acromion, the acromio-clavicular joint and the tip of the coracoid process. By applying pressure on the outer third of the clavicle and gradually moving laterally the acromio-clavicular joint can be palpated by the slight movement at the outer end of the clavicle. The acromion can easily be felt posteriorly and laterally to this joint. The tip of the coracoid process is most often felt less than two fingers' breadth below the lateral third of the clavicle. The joint space is usually lateral to it but occasionally may be slightly medial to it, depending on the tilt of the coracoid process.

TECHNIQUE

D URING THE DEVELOPMENT of the technique of arthrography to be described, varying amounts of dye were injected into the shoulders of fresh cadavera, not only to judge how much solution should be used to give the best detail on the roentgenograms but also to determine the capacity of the joint. In adults, the capacity varied from 28 to 35 cc. Strange as it may seem, some shoulders in women took more solution than comparable shoulders in men. In more than one instance, the right shoulder differed in capacity from the left by as much as 5 cc; this difference was more pronounced in cadavera over sixty years of age. This may be explained by the tendency of the capsule to contract in the shoulder which is used less habitually. In a normal joint it was found that the use of about 16 cc of solution resulted in roentgenograms with the best detail (See Figs. 4, 6, 8). When more than 16 cc was used, the shadow of the contrast medium became so dense that the outlines of the joint were obscured (See Figs. 5, 7, 9).

Another finding of interest was a communication between the joint proper and the subdeltoid bursa without evidence of a definite rupture. This was noted in four of the cadavera cases between the ages of sixty-five and seventy years. A similar finding was mentioned by Gassen (1902). It is known that a communication between the shoulder joint and the subdeltoid bursa may develop after a spontaneous rupture without any history of an injury. This occurs not infrequently in patients beyond the age of sixty years as the result of degenerative changes in the rotator cuff. This fact has been reported by other authors, especially Frostad. Dissection of the four shoulders with a communication between the joint and the bursa failed to establish definitely the cause of this communication. There was no evidence of a tear although in each

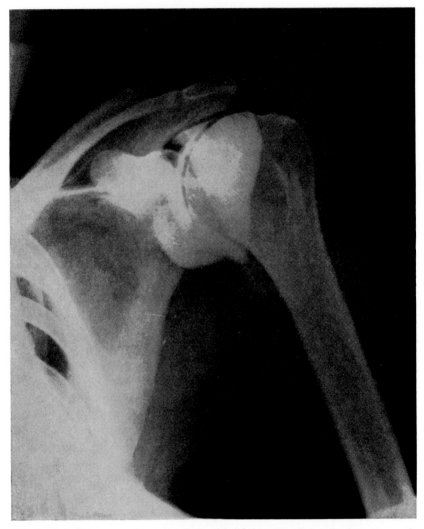

Figure 4. Arthrogram of a normal shoulder joint. Good detail when 16 cc of dye was injected.

instance the capsule posteriorly and superiorly was found to be rather thin, presumably due to attritional and degenerative changes. Incidentally, this communication was not seen until the joint had been fully distended with more than 28 cc of solution. Only then did the subdeltoid bursa become filled. It is possible

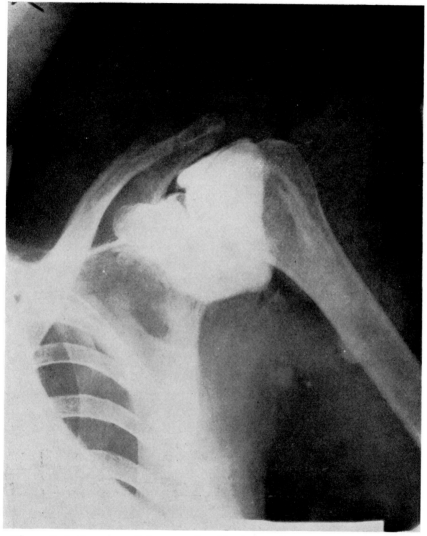

Figure 5. Arthrogram of the same shoulder injected with 25 cc of dye. Note less detail of the joint space and distension of biceps sheath by the dye.

that these openings could have been very minute in size not allowing the bursa to fill until the joint was under tension.

Our technique for injecting the contrast media varied depending to a great extent on the type of case with which we were dealing. We have used the anterior approach for most cases. In those

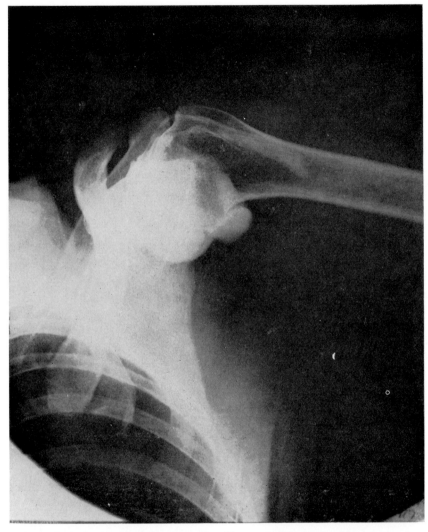

Figure 6. Arthrogram of the same shoulder as in Figure 4 with the arm in some abduction. Satisfactory outline of capsule and biceps sheath.

suspected of having an adhesive capsulitis or frozen shoulder, however, the posterior approach, at times, was found to be more satisfactory. One may ask why not use the posterior technique in all cases. The disadvantage is that the needle sometimes will bend when the patient is turned from the prone to the supine position

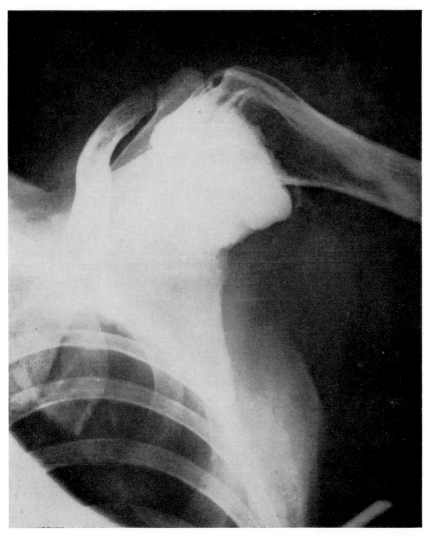

Figure 7. Same shoulder as in Figure 5 with arm in some abduction. Total of 25 cc of dye has been injected. Too much dye obscures the outline of the joint and also reveals the biceps sheath greatly distended and prolonged distally.

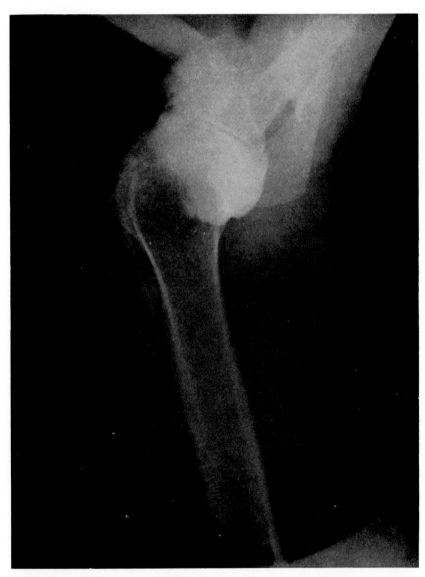

Figure 8. Axillary view of normal joint with 16 cc of dye injected. Note redundancy of the posterior capsule. The biceps sheath outlined anteriorly is partly overshadowed by the lesser tuberosity.

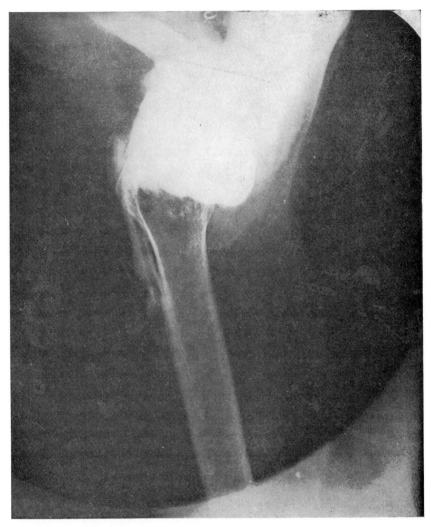

Figure 9. Axillary view after injection of 25 cc of dye. There is a poor out-line of the joint and lack of detail. The biceps sheath is also seen distended and prolonged downward.

to obtain axillary views. This has not been a real problem, but since each approach has proven satisfactory both will be described. The procedure is carried out in the Radiology Department using an image intensifier.

In the anterior approach, the patient is placed in the supine position with his arm by the side and in internal rotation. The shoulder is prepared using the usual sterile technique. The land-mark for injection is a point just below the tip of the coracoid process and slightly lateral to it. The site of injection is infiltrated with a local anesthetic including the deep tissues down to the neck of the scapula close to the glenoid. The volume of anesthetic used is between 10 and 15 cc depending on the size of the patient and their sensitivity to pain. A twenty gauge short beveled needle, two and a half or three inches long, is then inserted and directed straight toward the glenoid. When the bone is reached the needle is backed off slightly and then redirected a little more laterally so that it enters the joint space above the axillary fold (See Figs. 10 and 11). The position of the needle can now be checked by the use of the image intensifier unit. Originally a mixture of 12 cc of 35 percent Diodrast® and 4 cc of lidocaine was injected into the joint. Since Diodrast is no longer available, meglumine diatrizoate (Reno-M-60®) is now used. At first, a maximum of 2 cc is injected, and if the joint is well-outlined on the monitoring screen, the remainder of the solution is injected.

At times one will know immediately if the needle has been in-serted into the joint if synovial fluid emerges from the needle. Un-fortunately, this does not occur in shoulders with an adhesive capsulitis or rupture of the rotator cuff. By the very nature of the pathology of these conditions, very little if any joint fluid is pres-ent. Once we are certain that the joint has been entered all the dye is injected. Then the needle is quickly withdrawn and roent-genograms are taken immediately in the necessary positions. Since the dye is absorbed rather quickly it is necessary for the technician to obtain the films rapidly.

If one should encounter difficulty in inserting the needle, a helpful trick is to place the needle lateral to the joint space with the arm in external rotation so that the point of the needle rests on the humeral head. The arm is then rotated internally. When this is done, the point of the needle will tend to slip into the joint space. One may insert the needle directly into the joint either at its lower part (Fig. 12) or at its upper part (Fig. 13). In both lo-cations a satisfactory arthrogram will be obtained. Another method of locating the point of insertion of the needle is to view the joint

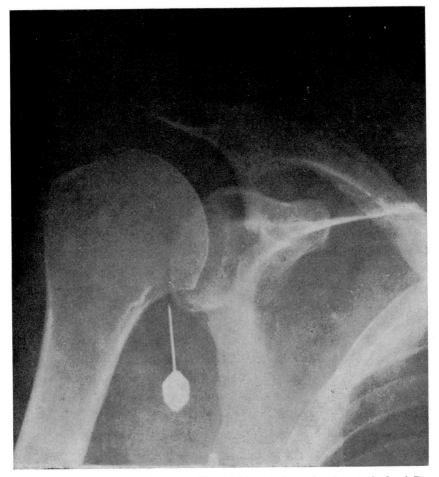

Figure 10. Shows needle in the axillary fold after inserting it anteriorly. A-P view. (Courtesy of *J. Bone Joint Surgery, 44-A:*1321, 1962.)

through the intensifying screen, mark the point of insertion on the skin with a marking pencil and then insert the needle through the point outlined on the skin.

We have found a twenty gauge needle to be the most satisfactory size since in postmortem cases it was observed that there was some leakage through the needle opening in the capsule if a larger gauge needle was used. Leakage of dye outside of the joint could easily confuse the interpretation of an arthrogram. A mixture of 12

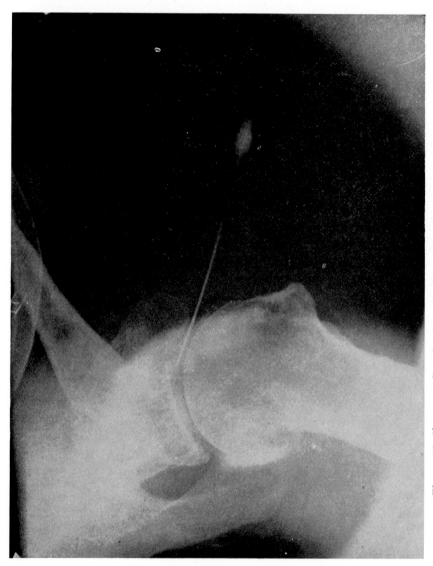

Figure 11. Shows needle placed in the joint through the anterior approach. Axillary view. (Courtesy of *J. Bone Joint Surgery, 44-A:1321,* 1962)

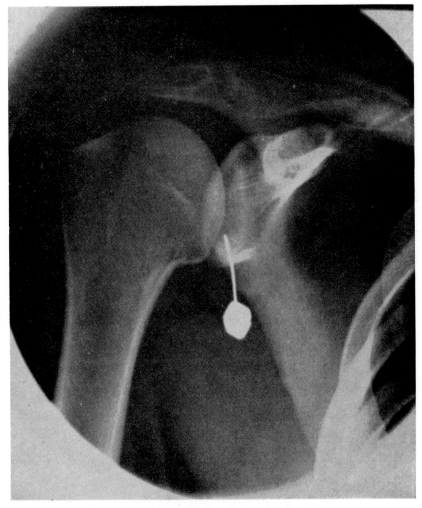

Figure 12. Needle inserted into the lower part of the joint.

cc of dye and 4 cc of 1 percent lidocaine eliminates any pain when the mixture is injected into the joint. If the solution should not be in the joint, the patient will have pain, but it will be less than that which results from the use of the dye without the added anesthetic.

The appearance of a normal arthrogram can be seen in Figures 4, 6 and 8. Figures 14 to 23 also show normal arthrograms. **It**

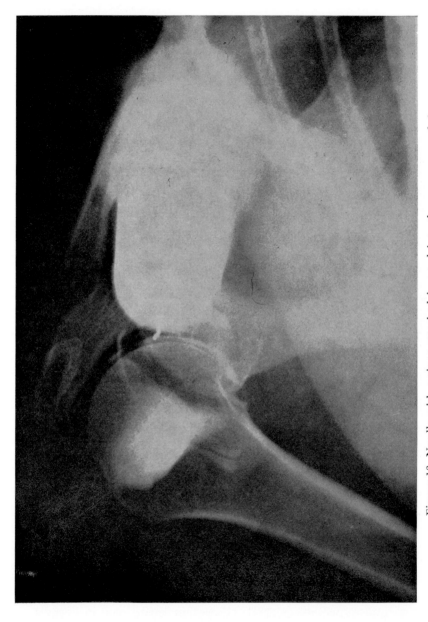

Figure 13. Needle with syringe attached inserted into the upper part of the joint.

should be noted that in some cases the subscapularis bursa is well-outlined (Fig. 14) while in others, it is somewhat smaller and is not visualized well (Fig. 15). This also applies to the bicipital sheath which is occasionally seen prolonged downward for some distance, while in other cases it is barely visible. A view taken with the arm in internal rotation (Fig. 16) has a different appearance than one taken with the arm in external rotation.

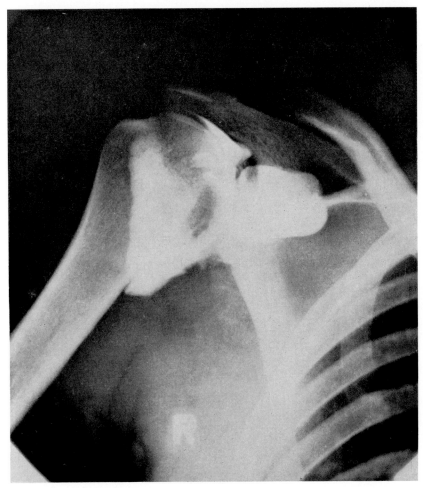

Figure 14. Arthrogram of a normal shoulder. Biceps sheath not visible but the subscapularis bursa is well outlined. A-P view with the arm in external rotation. (Courtesy of *J. Bone Joint Surgery, 44-A:*1321, 1962.)

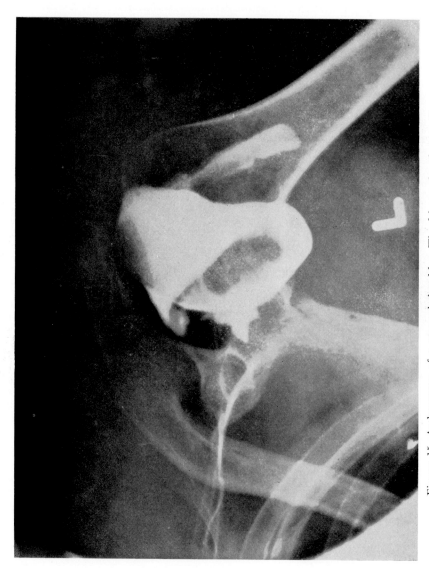

Figure 15. Arthrogram of a normal shoulder. The biceps sheath is well outlined but the subscapularis bursa is small. (Courtesy of *J. Bone Joint Surgery,* *44-A*:1321, 1962.)

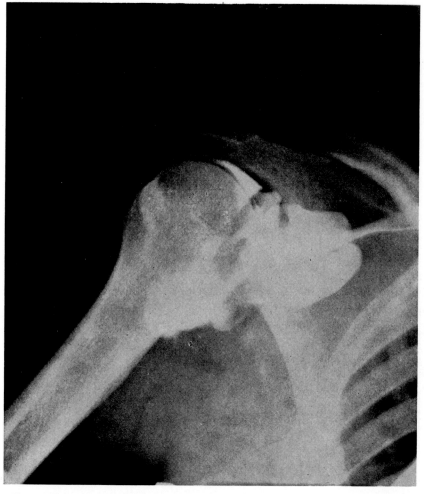

Figure 16. Arthrogram of the same shoulder as in Figure 14 but with the arm in internal rotation. (Courtesy of *J. Bone Joint Surgery, 44-A:*1321, 1962.)

When the arm is abducted the normal axillary fold is obliterated. This manuever is helpful in outlining the biceps sheath (Fig. 17). Often the biceps sheath is not outlined well with the arm at the side; but with the arm abducted, the dye is pushed superiorly by the obliteration of the reflected axillary fold and the solution runs into the synovial sheath of the biceps without difficulty. The axil-

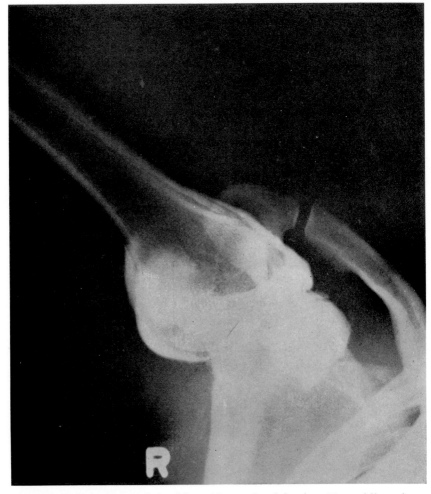

Figure 17. Arthrogram of shoulder with arm in abduction. Note obliteration of the axillary fold. Some dye is also seen in the biceps sheath. (Courtesy of *J. Bone Joint Surgery, 44-A:*1321, 1962.)

lary view (Fig. 18) is interesting because one can observe the outline of the subscapularis bursa anteriorly as well as the biceps sheath running over the lesser tuberosity. This view also reveals the relaxation or redundancy of the posterior capsule of the shoulder joint. This was found to be present in all normal shoulders. The view of the bicipital groove (Fig. 19) is taken by directing the tube along the longitudinal axis of the shaft of the humerus

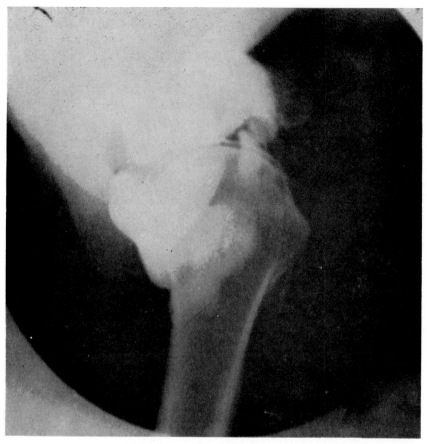

Figure 18. Axillary view. Note the redundancy of the posterior capsule of the joint. The subscapularis bursa is well-filled anterior to the neck of the scapula. (Courtesy of *J. Bone Joint Surgery, 44-A*:1321, 1962.)

with the film placed above the shoulder. This view reveals a circumferential outline of the sheath of the long head of the biceps tendon.

The posterior approach is occasionally used in cases of adhesive capsulitis or frozen shoulder. In this condition the capsule is contracted superiorly, anteriorly and inferiorly; hence it may be difficult to inject the dye into the joint anteriorly. In my earlier attempts at arthrography this was the cause of failure to obtain arthrograms of shoulders with an adhesive capsulitis. The posterior approach solved this difficulty. With some redundancy of

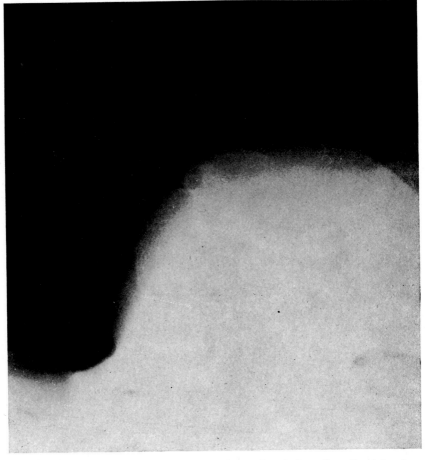

Figure 19. Bicipital groove view. The biceps sheath is well-outlined in the bicipital groove. (Courtesy of *J. Bone Joint Surgery, 44-A*:1321, 1962.)

the capsule posteriorly, the needle can be inserted with relative ease. In this approach the patient lies prone with his arm by his side and in internal rotation. A good landmark for injection is a slight depression felt just below the medial portion of the acromion where it joins the spine of the scapula in a direct line posteriorly from the tip of the coracoid process. A twenty gauge needle is inserted under sterile precautions, using local anesthesia, directed slightly upward so that the needle enters the upper part of the joint (Fig. 20). The position of the needle is checked by

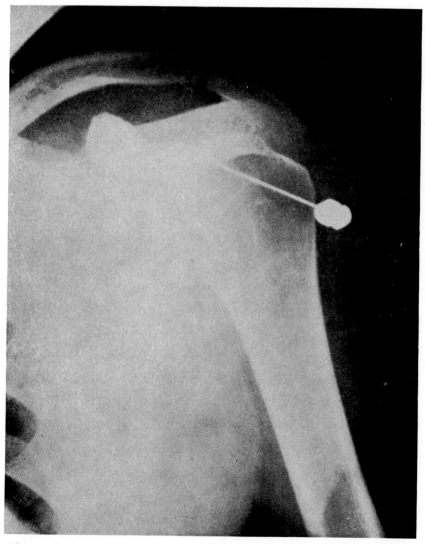

Figure 20. Posterior-anterior roentgenogram of a right shoulder showing needle inserted posteriorly into the upper part of the joint. (Courtesy of *J. Bone Joint Surgery, 44-A:*1321, 1962.)

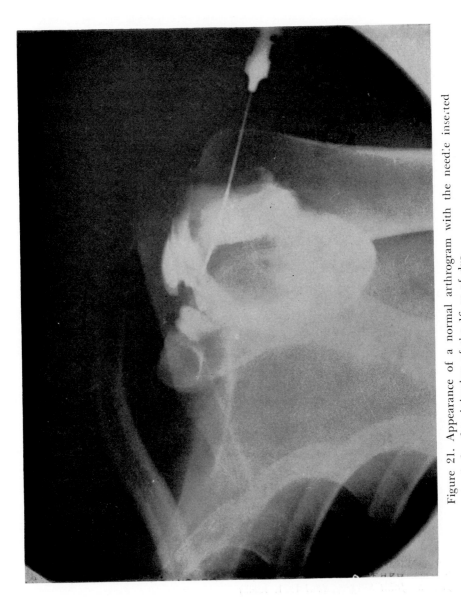

Figure 21. Appearance of a normal arthrogram with the needle inserted posteriorly after injection of the 16 cc of dye.

fluroscopic control and, if the instillation of 2 cc of dye shows that the fluid is in the joint, the remainder of the dye can then be injected. The desired roentgenograms are made immediately (Fig. 21). The arthrograms taken in the posterior-anterior plane (Figs. 22 and 23) have a different appearance than those taken in the anterior-posterior projection.

As mentioned, the ideal amount to be injected is 16 cc of solution (12 cc of dye and 4 cc of 1% lidocaine). This can be done easily without any resistance to the plunger of the syringe. If there should be resistance the injection should be discontinued, as this can mean only one of two things; either the needle has not been placed correctly in the joint or one is dealing with a case of

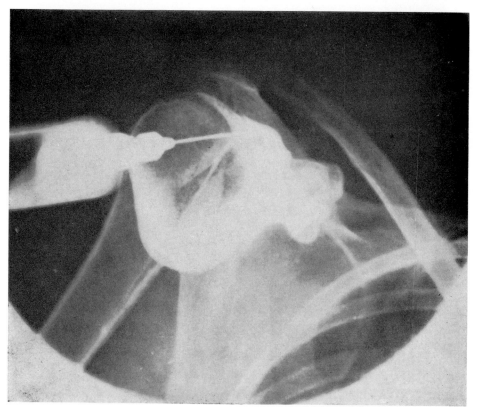

Figure 22. Dye being injected into a left shoulder from behind. Joint is well-outlined as is the subscapularis bursa.

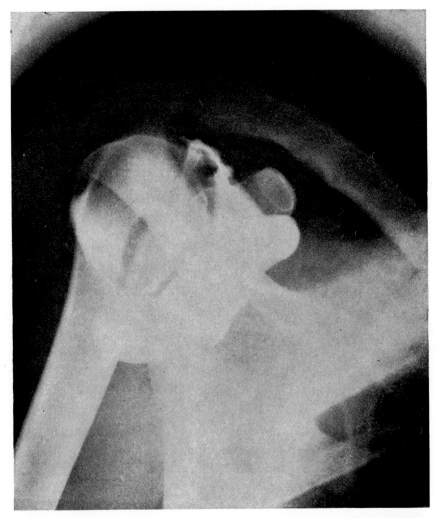

Figure 23. Normal arthrogram of a left shoulder taken in the posterior-anterior position. Note the well outlined dependent axillary fold, the subscapularis bursa as well as the biceps sheath. (Courtesy of *J. Bone Joint Surgery, 44-A:*1321, 1962.)

adhesive capsulitis. In the latter instance, where the joint capacity is only about 5 to 10 cc further attempts to inject dye under pressure may cause the solution to rupture through the subscapularis bursa or the biceps sheath. This may obscure the interpretation of the arthrogram or give a false appearance of a tear of the rotator cuff.

Other approaches to the shoulder joint have been used besides the routine anterior or posterior approaches. The former is more ideal as the needle can be placed in the upper, middle or lower part of the joint, even in the dependent axillary fold and one can still obtain good arthrograms. Insertion of the needle superiorly

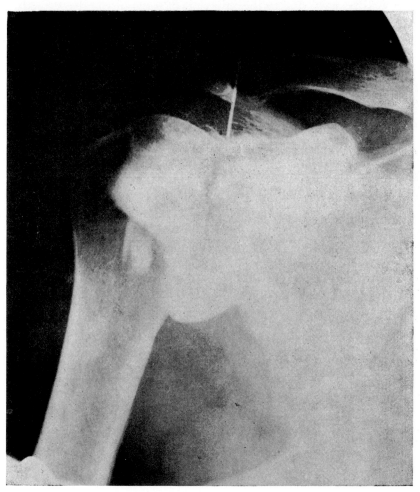

Figure 24. Normal arthrogram using the superior approach through the acromio-clavicular joint. An excellent outline of the shoulder joint is obtained.

through the acromio-clavicular joint has been performed and a satisfactory study resulted (Fig. 24).

The needle can also be inserted from the lateral side of the
shoulder, placing it horizontally just below the acromion. One
must be sure he has entered the joint always using a short beveled
needle. Otherwise, the opening in the needle will be half in and
half out of the joint and, after instillation of the dye, a false rupture will be seen, due to the injection of some of the dye directly

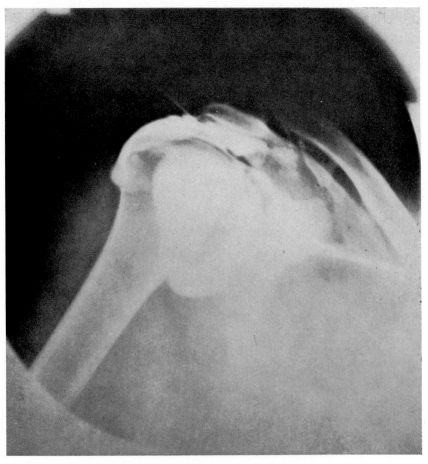

Figure 25. Arthrogram gives the appearance of a false rupture. Dye partly in
the subdeltoid bursa and the remainder in the joint due to the use of a
long beveled needle which is half in and half out of the joint.

into the subdeltoid bursa and the remainder into the joint cavity (Fig. 25).

Any surgeon or radiologist who is reluctant to expose his hands under the intensifying screen can try the technique utilized by my son, Jules. He uses a small plastic tubing about 50 cm long between the needle and syringe connected by adapters. Eighteen cc of solution is used to compensate for the 2 cc of dye which remains in the tubing after injecting 16 cc of the solution into the joint. Sterile venous or anesthesia extension sets are now available and serve the same purpose admirably (Figs. 26 and 27). This procedure has two other advantages. The needle with the tubing at-

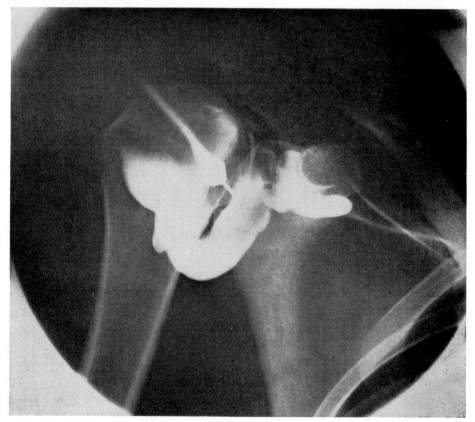

Figure 26. Arthrogram outlines the joint well using a plastic extension tubing between the needle and syringe.

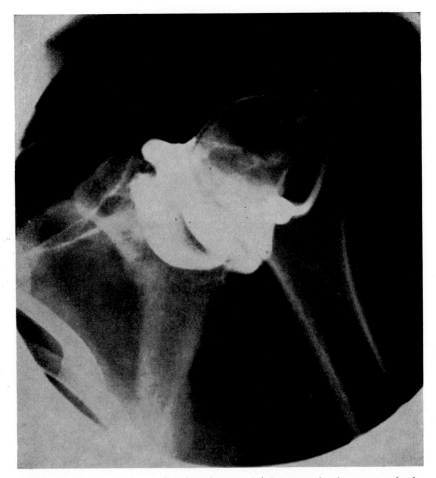

Figure 27. An arthrogram showing decreased joint capacity in a case of ad-hesive capsulitis. The hub of the needle is attached to a venous extension tube.

tached can be left in the joint and, if insufficient dye has not been instilled, additional dye can be added. If any of the films should turn out poorly due to improper technique, more dye can be injected if some has been absorbed in the interval.

If there is any doubt in the interpretation of the arthrograms one may perform bilateral examinations. Any variations from the normal found in the involved side will help to determine the pathologic process present in that joint.

Chapter Three

ADHESIVE CAPSULITIS

ADHESIVE CAPSULITIS or the so-called "frozen shoulder" is probably the most common shoulder lesion encountered in the middle-aged. Literature is replete with a vast amount of confusing and contradictory information over the etiology, pathology and treatment. The arthrographic findings in this condition confirm many of the pathological findings previously reported. Arthrograms have also demonstrated the healing of the capsule after manipulation of the shoulder under general anesthesia, as well as the location of the tear at the dependent axillary fold of the joint. Arthrography has proven of great help in differentiating between a case of stiff and painful shoulder and one of a true adhesive capsulitis.

The essential lesion is a chronic inflammatory process involving the capsule of the shoulder causing a thickening and contracture of this structure which secondarily becomes adherent to the humeral head. In addition, adhesions are discernible at the reflected fold of the capsule distal to the anatomical neck of the humerus (Fig. 28). As a result of this thickening and contracture, the capacity of the shoulder joint in adhesive capsulitis is reduced to 5 to 10 cc. Occasionally, the subscapularis bursa and the biceps sheath may be involved and will not be visualized by arthrography.

The following case reports demonstrate the changes which can take place in shoulders with an adhesive capsulitis:

M.S., a thirty-nine-year-old female, gave a history of having persistent pain in the left shoulder for about eight months. Exercises and mild manipulations had given her no relief. When examined, active abduction of the shoulder was 90 degrees and passive abduction was 95 degrees. Upon internal rotation, the left hand reached the left buttock. Arthrograms were made of both shoulders. The right shoulder easily

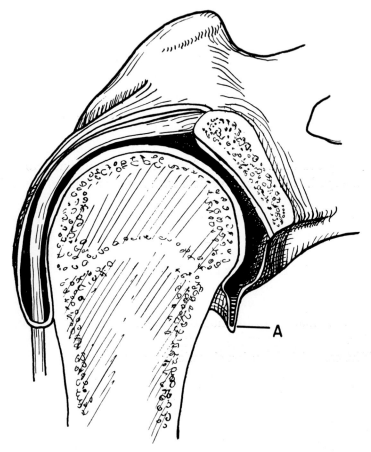

Figure 28. A vertical section through the shoulder joint showing (A) the adhesion of the reflected dependent fold of the capsule. (Courtesy of *J. Bone Joint Surgery, 27:*211, 1945.)

took the 16 cc of solution that was injected and the arthrograms (Figs. 29 to 31) were normal. The left shoulder only took 10 cc of solution and the arthrograms (Figs. 32 to 34) revealed a definite decrease in joint capacity with almost complete obliteration of the axillary fold. The subscapularis bursa, as well as the bicipital sheath, were not visualized. In this case, it appeared that the inflammatory process had obliterated the subscapularis bursa and tendon sheath since even with abduction of the arm the picture did not change. Axillary views of the two shoulders and the anterior-posterior views emphasizes the excellent

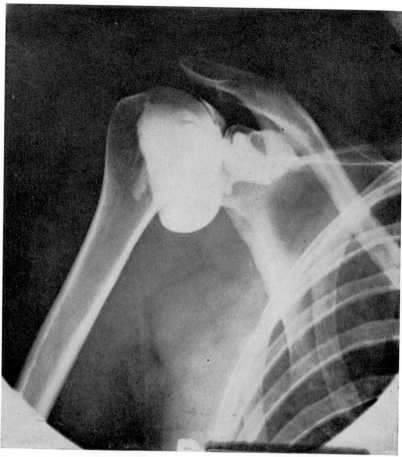

Figure 29. Arthrogram of the right shoulder is normal. The axillary fold is well outlined and the biceps sheath can be seen easily. (Courtesy of *J. Bone Joint Surgery, 44-A*:1321, 1962.)

outline of the subscapularis bursa, the bicipital sheath and the loose capsule of the right shoulder, which is normal when compared with the decreased joint capacity and obliteration of the dependent axillary fold in the left shoulder with an adhesive capsulitis.

During the original investigative study on frozen shoulders some patients were operated upon to clarify certain controversial points. Where would the capsule tear when closed manipulation

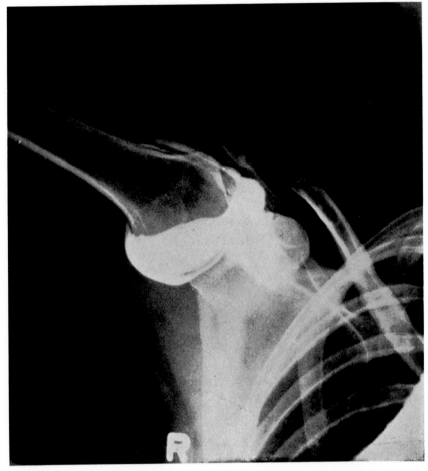

Figure 30. Arthrogram of the right shoulder with the arm in abduction. The axillary fold has become tense and dye can be seen in the subscapularis bursa and biceps sheath. (Courtesy of *J. Bone Joint Surgery, 44-A:*1321, 1962.)

was done on the shoulder? After obtaining a complete exposure of the shoulder joint by turning down the conjoined tendons of the short head of the biceps tendon and coracobrachialis these shoulders were manipulated under direct vision. It was observed that the capsule would invariably tear at the reflected fold near the base of the neck of the humerus (Fig. 35). This was a constant finding.

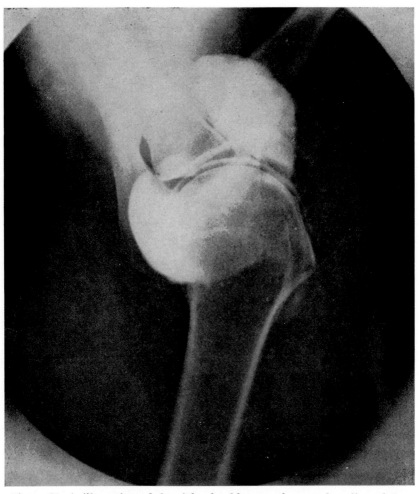

Figure 31. Axillary view of the right shoulder reveals a good outline of the subscapularis bursa and biceps sheath. Note the relaxation of the posterior capsule of the joint. (Courtesy of *J. Bone Joint Surgery, 44-A:*1321, 1962.)

Five weeks later the patient's left shoulder was manipulated under general anesthesia. Arthrography was performed just prior to the manipulation while the patient was under anesthesia. The findings were the same as shown in Figures 32 and 34. Roentgenograms were made immediately after the manipulation. They revealed that the capsule had torn at the adherent axillary fold with escape of the dye into the axillary space and inferiorly along the inner aspect of the humerus (Figs. 36, 37). Under the usual post manipulation care the patient

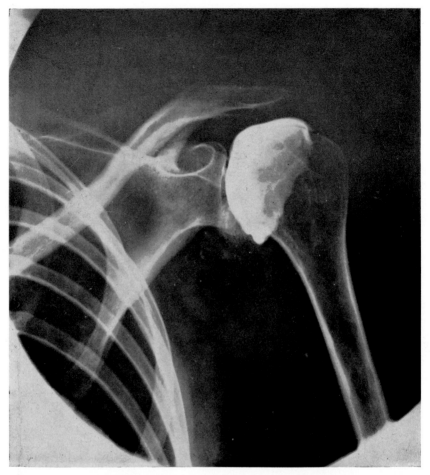

Figure 32. Arthrogram demonstrates the findings seen in adhesive capsulitis. There is a decreased joint capacity with complete obliteration of the axillary fold. The subscapularis bursa and biceps sheath are not outlined. (Courtesy of *J. Bone Joint Surgery, 44-A*:1321, 1962.)

did quite well, regaining 180 degrees of active and passive abduction within a month after the manipulation.

Although this patient regained satisfactory function of the left shoulder in a very short period of time, she started to complain of pain in the right shoulder. Over five weeks time she gradually lost motion so that she could only abduct to 120 degrees and upon internal rotation the right hand only touched the right buttock. The left shoulder continued to have an excellent range of motion without pain. Arthrograms

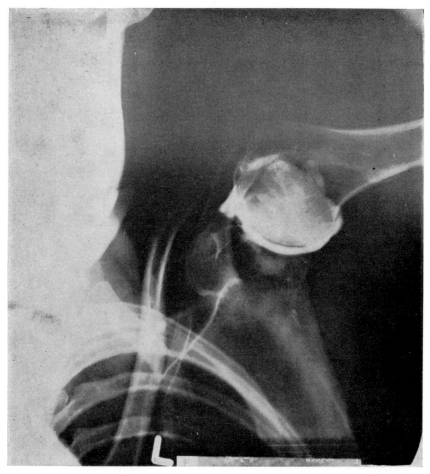

Figure 33. Arthrogram of case of adhesive capsulitis with the arm in maximum abduction. (Courtesy of *J. Bone Joint Surgery, 44-A:*1321, 1962.)

were repeated on both shoulders two and one-half months following the manipulation of the left shoulder. At that time only 6 cc of dye could be injected into the right shoulder which three and one-half months previously had easily taken 16 cc. The arthrogram of this shoulder showed definite evidence of an adhesive capsulitis with decreased joint capacity, obliteration of the axillary fold and almost complete lack of filling of the subscapularis bursa (Figs. 38, 39). With the arm in abduction the arthrogram showed no significant change. The left shoulder, which had been manipulated ten weeks earlier, appeared almost normal by arthrogram with a good axillary fold which tensed

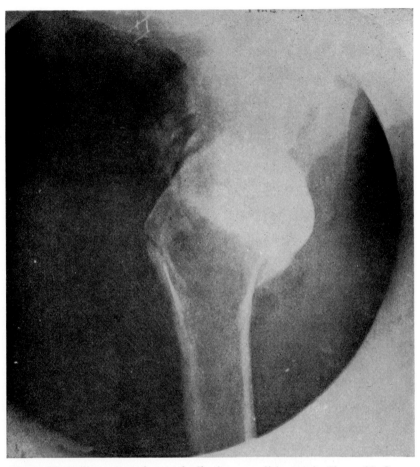

Figure 34. Axillary view of case of adhesive capsulitis seen in Figure 32. Compare with the normal shoulder in Figure 31. (Courtesy of *J. Bone Joint Surgery, 44-A*:1321, 1962.)

in abduction (Figs. 40, 41). The axillary view outlined the biceps sheath and the normal appearance of the posterior capsule (Fig. 42).

The right shoulder was manipulated under general anesthesia two weeks later. Arthrograms were also obtained during the manipulative procedure and they revealed the same changes that were observed after manipulation of the left shoulder, i.e. tearing of the capsule at the adherent axillary fold and escape of the dye into the axillary space and along the inner side of the humerus (Figs. 43, 44). In three months this patient had good range of motion in the right shoulder with no pain.

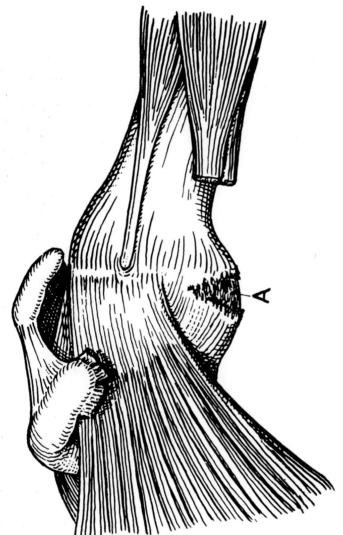

Figure 35. Tearing of the capsule at the dependent axillary fold (A) near the base of the neck of the humerus during manipulation. (Courtesy of A.A.O.S. *Instructional Course Lectures, 6:281,* 1949.)

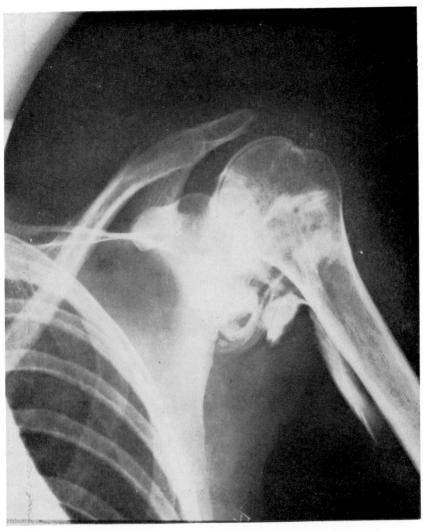

Figure 36. Arthrogram of the shoulder following manipulation of the arm under anesthesia. Note escape of dye at the site of tear in the adherent axillary fold. Dye extravasates into the axillary space and along the inner side of the arm. (Courtesy of *J. Bone Joint Surgery, 44-A*:1321, 1962.)

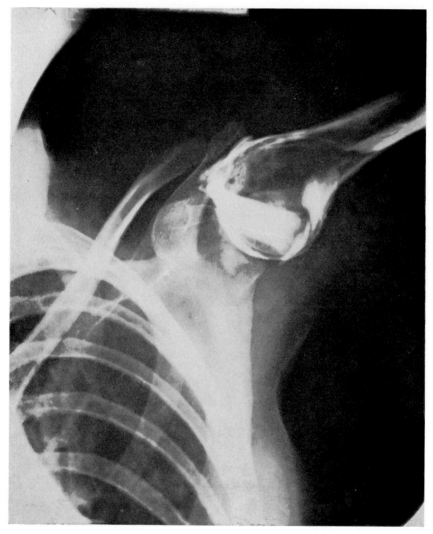

Figure 37. Arthrogram made after manipulation with the arm in abduction. (Courtesy of *J. Bone Joint Surgery, 44-A*:1321, 1962.)

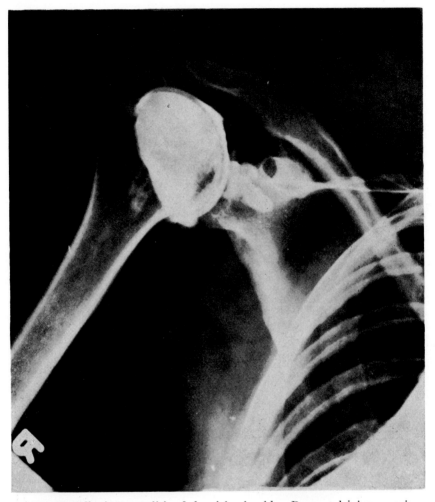

Figure 38. Adhesive capsulitis of the right shoulder. Decreased joint capacity and almost complete absence of the axillary fold. Compare with Figure 29 taken three and one half months earlier. (Courtesy of *J. Bone Joint Surgery, 44-A:*1321, 1962.)

The appearance of the arthrograms in patients with adhesive capsulitis may vary:

G. L., a fifty-one-year-old female, had pain in her left shoulder for more than six months. In addition to her limitation of motion she had

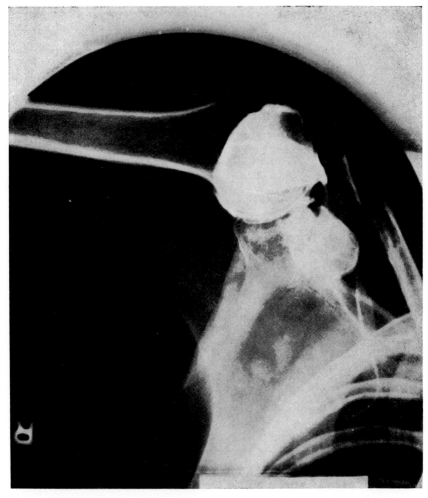

Figure 39. Arthrogram of shoulder when the arm is in maximum abduction. Compare with Figure 30. (Courtesy of *J. Bone Joint Surgery, 44-A*:1321, 1962.)

difficulty sleeping at night because of the pain. Active abduction was only 80 degrees and upon internal rotation she could only reach her buttock with her left hand. The arthrogram revealed definite decrease in joint capacity, no visualization of the biceps sheath and obliteration of the dependent axillary fold (Fig. 45). At the time of arthrography the joint accepted only 5 cc of dye. The shoulder was manipulated under general anesthesia. Following the manipulation the left arm

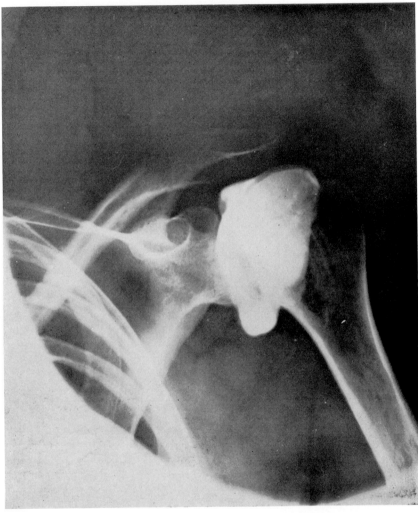

Figure 40. Arthrogram of the left shoulder performed a little over two months after manipulation under general anesthesia. Note normal appearing axillary fold. Compare with Figures 32 and 33. (Courtesy of *J. Bone Joint Surgery*, *44-A*:1321, 1962.)

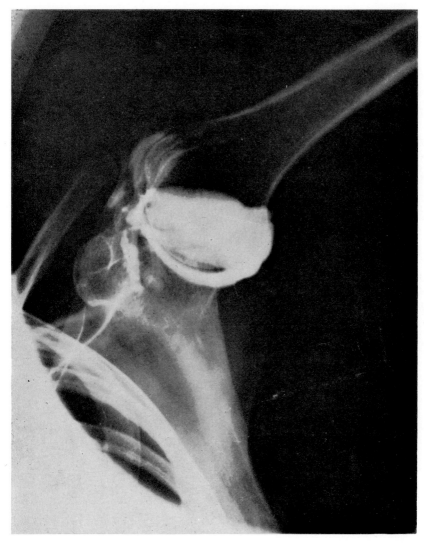

Figure 41. Arthrogram made with the arm in abduction. The axillary fold becomes tense. Observe some dye in the biceps sheath. (Courtesy of *J. Bone Joint Surgery, 44-A:*1321, 1962.)

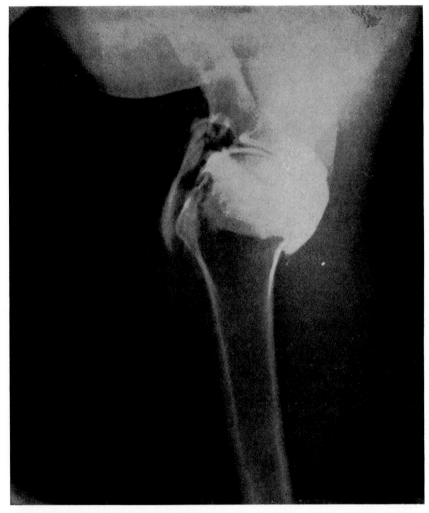

Figure 42. The axillary view outlines the biceps sheath and shows the normal relaxation of the posterior capsule. Compare with Figure 34. (Courtesy of *J. Bone Joint Surgery, 44-A:*1321, 1962.)

was tied to the head of the bed at 90 degrees of abduction by a swathe. Abduction, external and internal rotation exercises were encouraged while in bed. She was discharged from the hospital five days after the manipulation and continued to be observed in the office where she received physical therapy treatments to the shoulder. The patient was instructed in regular abduction and rotation exercises which were to

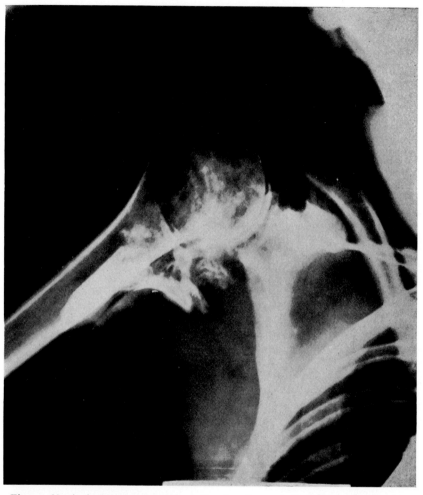

Figure 43. Arthrogram taken immediately after manipulation of the right shoulder. Dye escaping through the tear in the axillary fold. (Courtesy of *J. Bone Joint Surgery, 44-A*:1321, 1962.)

be done at home. After three and one-half months she had good range of motion in the shoulder with only a slight amount of discomfort. An arthrogram done at that time revealed a normal axillary fold and 16 cc of dye was easily instilled into the joint (Fig. 46).

In another case of adhesive capsulitis, the needle was inserted in lower portion of the joint anteriorly but above the dependent axillary fold (Fig. 47). Note that the arm is in internal rotation to facilitate

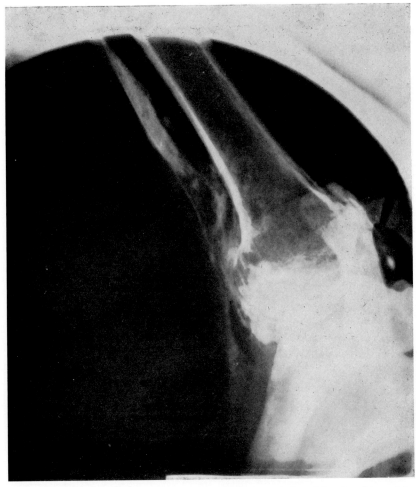

Figure 44. Arthrogram taken after manipulation of the right shoulder with the arm in abduction. Dye is seen extravasating along the inner side of the arm. (Courtesy of *J. Bone Joint Surgery, 44-A:*1321, 1962.)

insertion of the needle. The joint took only 8.5 cc of dye. Although the biceps sheath is outlined, the subscapularis bursa and the dependent axillary fold are poorly visualized (Fig. 48). Figure 49 demonstrates the escape of dye from the dependent axillary fold after manipulation of the shoulder in abduction and external rotation.

E. H., a forty-eight-year-old female, was referred because of pain in the right shoulder which had gradually evolved over a period of six

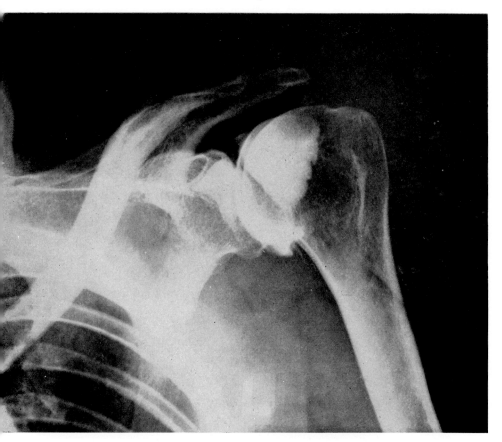

Figure 45. Arthrogram of patient with an adhesive capsulitis. Only 5 cc of dye could be injected into the joint. Note obliteration of the axillary fold and biceps sheath.

months. She could not sleep on her right side and she had difficulty hooking her bras and tying her apron strings. Active abduction was only sixty degrees and upon internal rotation she could barely reach two inches below her belt line. At arthrography the needle was inserted posteriorly but the joint only took 7 cc of dye (Fig. 50). Despite the contracture of the capsule the biceps sheath was visualized in the posterior-anterior projection (Fig. 51). After removal of the needle the patient was turned to the supine position and a roentgenogram taken in the anterior-posterior projection. The arthrogram reveals the absence of the axillary fold but excellent outline of the biceps sheath (Fig. 52).

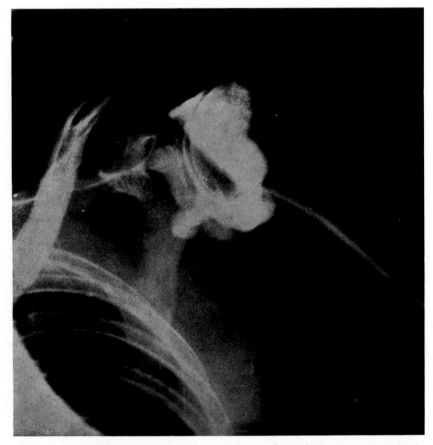

Figure 46. Arthrogram of the left shoulder performed three and one half months after manipulation. Sixteen cc of dye could be injected into the joint. Normal axillary fold is present.

There is an occasional case of adhesive capsulitis where one may not feel any real resistance to the plunger of the syringe when instilling the dye into the joint. In these instances one may get the impression that the joint will take the entire 16 cc of solution. However, if one will observe the joint closely on the monitor during the procedure one will see that most of the fluid has ruptured through the subscapularis bursa and has extravasated into the soft tissues medially. Very little dye is present in the joint proper and the humeral head is not completely covered by the solution (Figs.

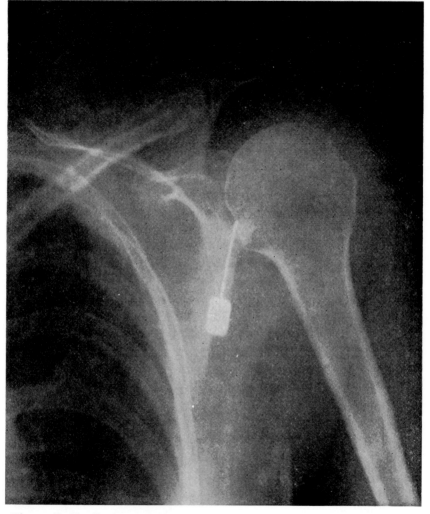

Figure 47. Needle inserted anteriorly in the lower portion of the joint just above the dependent axillary fold.

53, 54) . Only through experience can the surgeon learn the feel of the slightest resistance to the plunger. When this occurs no further attempt should be made to instill dye.

Figure 55 shows the arthrogram of a female, age fifty-three years, with an adhesive capsulitis. The needle was placed in the joint su-

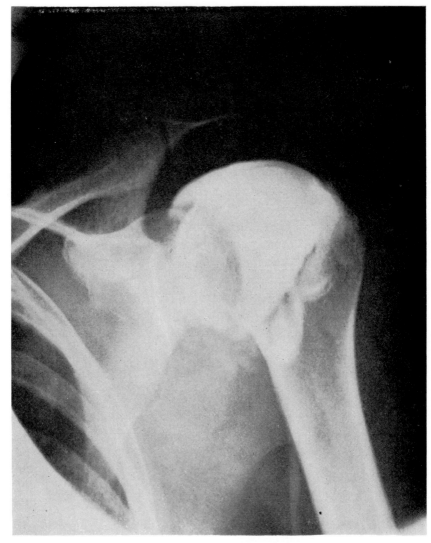

Figure 48. Arthrogram is indicative of an adhesive capsulitis. The dependent axillary fold and the subscapularis bursa are poorly outlined.

periorly above the adherent dependent axillary fold. After only 7 cc of dye had been injected when resistance was felt to the plunger. Note the decreased joint capacity and the absence of the dependent fold.

In the treatment of a so-called frozen shoulder there is the problem of differentiating between patients with a true adhesive cap-

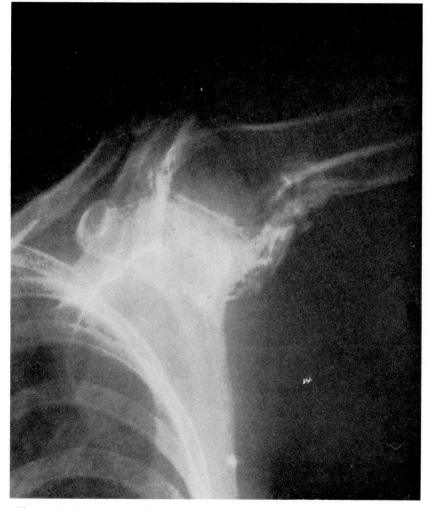

Figure 49. Note escape of dye from the axillary fold after manipulation of the arm under general anesthesia.

sulitis and those with a stiff and painful shoulder in which the limitation of motion is due primarily to muscle spasm. Limitation due to muscle spasm not infrequently follows some form of trauma or tendinitis. Since the clinical findings of both types are essentially the same, arthrography can be used not only as a valuable diagnostic tool but also as a therapeutic aid. The arthrographic picture of a case of stiff and painful shoulder will be simi-

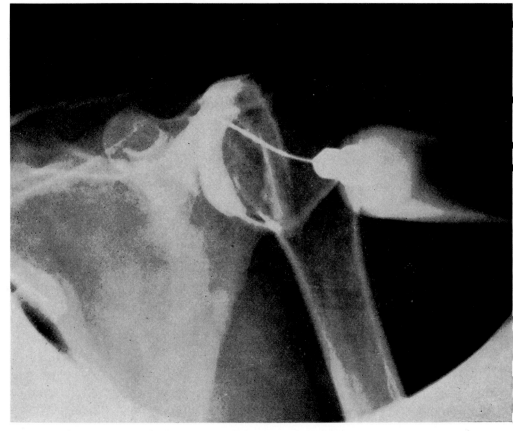

Figure 50. Case of adhesive capsulitis of the right shoulder. Dye injected into the joint posteriorly. Only 7 cc could be instilled into the joint.

lar to that of a normal shoulder. The capsule is not contracted and the axillary fold is not adherent to itself (Fig. 56). The treatment of a stiff and painful shoulder is conservative, namely physical therapy and increasing active exercises for the arm. Injections of a steroid with a local anesthetic at times may also be used.

An infrequent cause of stiff and painful shoulder is a hemarthrosis of the shoulder joint. Suggesting arthrography was of value in making a definite diagnosis in the following cases:

A female, thirty-one years of age, working as a maid in a hotel caught her hand in a door as it was closing. She not only injured her

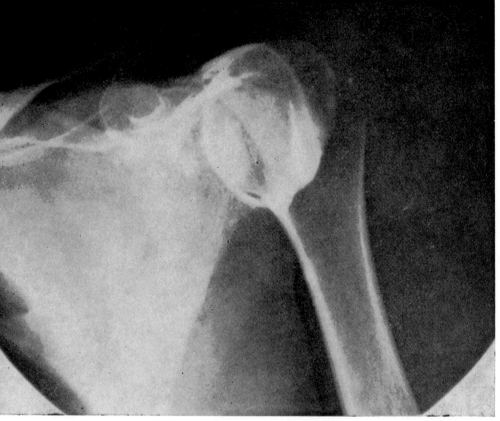

Figure 51. Appearance of the arthrogram viewed in the posterior-anterior projection after removal of the needle from the joint as seen in Figure 50.

middle fingers but also felt a pull in her right shoulder with subsequent pain. The bruises of her fingers cleared up in ten days but the pain and stiffness in her shoulder persisted. Active abduction was 120 degrees and passive abduction was 135 degrees. External rotation was 60 degrees, while on internal rotation she could not touch the belt line. Three possibilities were considered. The patient had either an adhesive capsulitis, a possible rupture of the rotator cuff or a stiff and painful shoulder. When the needle was inserted into the shoulder joint when performing arthrography, blood gushed out of the needle and a total of 24 cc of blood was removed from the joint. Following this procedure the patient was able to move her shoulder freely with very little discomfort.

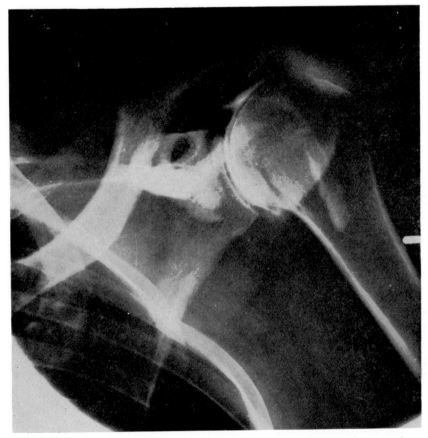

Figure 52. Arthrogram of the right shoulder taken in the anterior-posterior view. Note the excellent outline of the biceps sheath but a poor outline of the subscapularis bursa and obliteration of the dependent axillary fold.

A young man, twenty years of age, had an anterior dislocation of his right shoulder reduced three weeks previously. Following removal of the Velpeau dressings he had continued pain with definite limitation in abduction. At the time of insertion of the needle for an arthrogram, 18 cc of blood was removed. The pain rapidly disappeared and the patient regained full motion in the shoulder.

In an adhesive capsulitis the arthrograms will show a decrease in joint capacity and adherence of the reflected dependent fold as a result of the contracture and thickening of the capsule (Fig. 57).

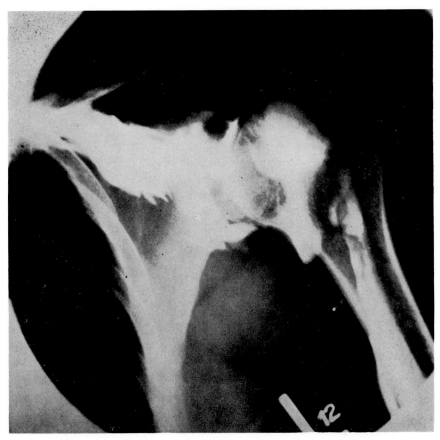

Figure 53. Case of adhesive capsulitis. Note escape of dye through the subscapularis bursa and the biceps sheath as the result of forcing all the dye into the joint.

The biceps sheath is outlined well as it is in the majority of cases of adhesive capsulitis, thus confirming the fact that a biceps tenosynovitis or tendinitis is one of the end results of adhesive capsulitis and not its cause. Figure 58 again demonstrates a good outline of the biceps sheath in another case of adhesive capsulitis.

A brief outline of the treatment of patients with an adhesive capsulitis might be appropriate. The cases can be grouped into three categories regardless of the age, sex or duration of the disease:

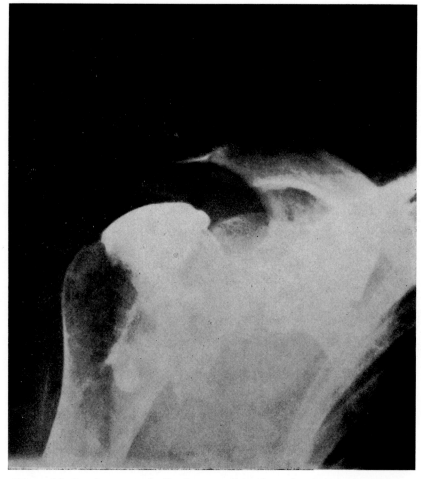

Figure 54. Another case of adhesive capsulitis where the dye was forced into the joint beyond its capacity causing the solution to escape through the subscapularis bursa. Note the irregularity at the distal portion of the biceps sheath as well as an uncomplete filling of the sheath suggestive of a biceps tenosynovitis.

1. This group consists of patients who can abduct more than 90 degrees and whose joint capacity by arthrography may vary from 10 to 12 cc. Such patients can be given physical therapy followed by exercises and gentle manipulations in abduction and external rotation. After a period of three to six months the majority of the

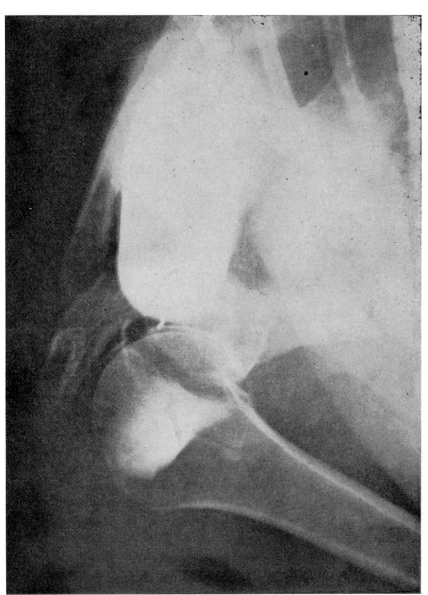

Figure 55. Shoulder joint capacity was only 7 cc. When resistance was felt to the plunger no further dye was instilled.

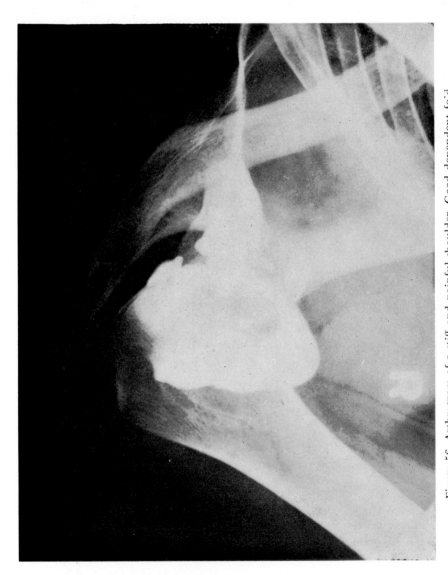

Figure 56. Arthrogram of a stiff and painful shoulder. Good dependent fold and subscapularis bursa well outlined. Normal arthrogram even though the biceps sheath is not visualized well.

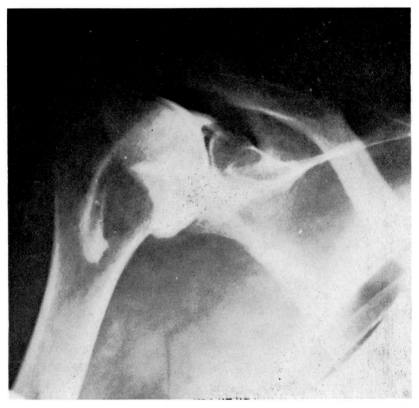

Figure 57. Arthrogram of a shoulder with an adhesive capsulitis. Decreased joint capacity, absent dependent axillary fold yet the biceps sheath is easily seen.

patients will have a good range of motion with a pain free shoulder joint. A similar form of treatment can be instituted for those patients with a stiff and painful shoulder although their recovery period is generally much shorter, good painless motion being obtained in three to eight weeks. I have yet to see a patient with a stiff and painful shoulder that required a manipulation under general anesthesia.

2. The second category for treatment is for those patients who have less than 90 degrees of abduction. Their joint capacity by arthrography may vary from 5 to 10 cc. These patients should have their shoulders manipulated under general anesthesia. The

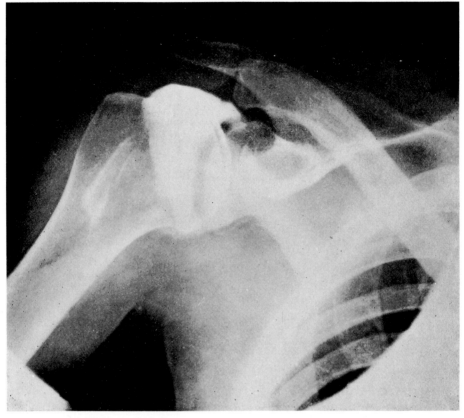

Figure 58. Another case of adhesive capsulitis. The arthrogram demonstrates a good outline of the biceps sheath.

results by this procedure have been quite good but the postmanipulative care must be carefully supervised. A patient who has had a shoulder manipulation under general anesthesia must be encouraged to exercise the arm in abduction and external rotation frequently. Most patients are very reluctant to perform these exercises on the first or second day after manipulation because of the initial pain, but the surgeon has to stress the fact that as one increases his motion by the exercises the pain will in turn decrease. After discharge from the hospital, generally in about five days, the patient must sleep with the arm held in about 90 degrees of ab-

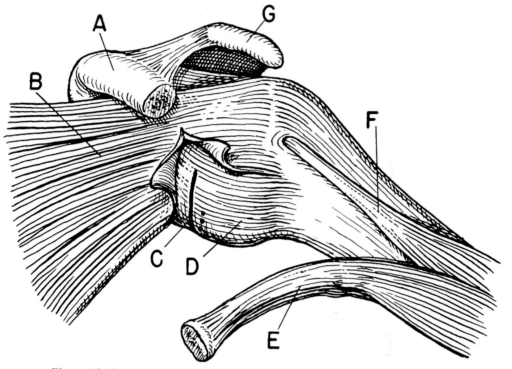

Figure 59. Exposure of the lower and inferior portion of the capsule (D) by cutting the inferior half of the subscapularis (B). Osteotomy of the coracoid process (A) or cutting the conjoined tendon of the short head of the biceps and coracobrachialis (E) to visualize the capsule. Acromion (G) and the long head of the biceps (F) is also seen. (Courtesy of *A.A.O.S. Instructional Course Lectures, 6*:281, 1949.)

duction by a swathe or towel tied to the head of the bed for about two weeks. Supervised physical therapy and persistent exercises for the shoulder will, as a rule, produce a useful arm with little or no pain in two or four months.

3. The third category of patients will require intervention by an arthrotomy at the anterior-inferior portion of the dependent axillary fold (Fig. 59). This group of patients generally comprise those which have been difficult to handle in the past. There are four indications:

a. Cases which recur after a manipulation under anesthesia.

b. Those which result from a dislocation of the shoulder. Certainly any attempt to manipulate such shoulders under anesthesia can result in another dislocation.

c. Those resulting from fractures of the surgical neck of the humerus. Any attempt at a manipulation could result in another fracture.

d. Those cases of adhesive capsulitis which reveal definite bone atrophy by roentgenograms.

Since a manipulation under general anesthesia of any of the four described types of cases lend themselves to risk to the bone structure or joint, an arthrotomy at the dependent axillary fold, the site of pathology, is the procedure of choice. The shoulder is exposed through the anterior axillary approach. Once the capsule has been incised it can be separated from the humeral head by the use of the curved separators seen in Figures 60 and 61. This operation was first described in the Instructional Course Lectures of the American Academy of Orthopedic Surgeons (1949). Two modifications have been made in the procedure. If it was necessary to detach the conjoined tendon of the short head of the biceps and coracobrachialis, the coracoid was not osteotomized, but was sectioned about 1 cm distal to the tip of the coracoid. When closing the wound it was easier to resuture the conjoined tendon ends together rather than using a screw to hold the coracoid fragment in place. The healing time was also lessened. The separator with the small tip, seen in the middle of the photograph in Figure 60, was found to be very useful. It is inserted into the cut capsule to gain access into the joint allowing easier use of the other two separators.

The aftercare is essentially the same as outlined for the patients who have had their shoulder manipulated under general anesthesia. What has impressed me most about the operation was that all patients, upon their discharge from the hospital, had almost complete relief from the persistent pain that had existed prior to the operation. This could be due to the release of capsular tension about the humeral head. With relief of pain the patients were willing to move their arms more freely, and they invariably obtained satisfactory range of motion in two or three months. This fact alone could make the operation worthwhile.

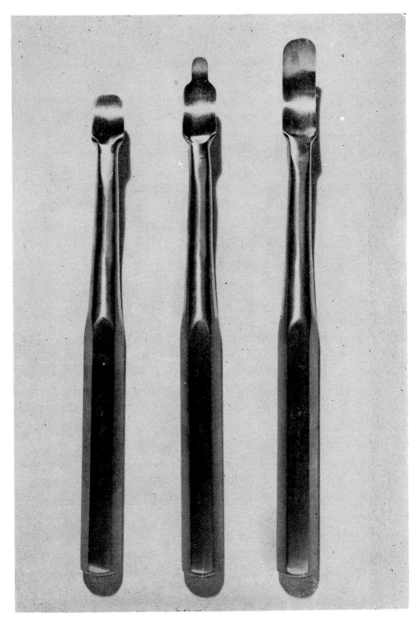

Figure 60. Front view of the three instruments used to separate the contracted capsule from the humeral head.

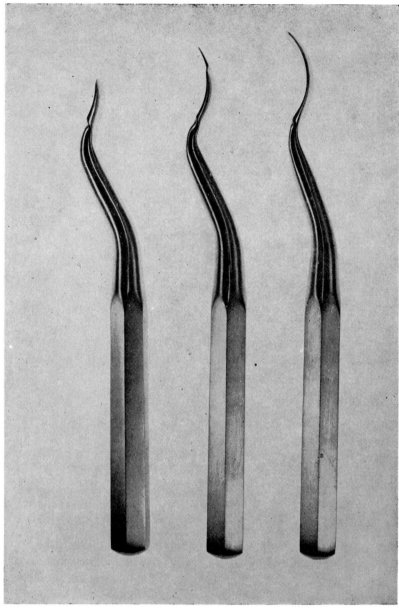

Figure 61. Side view of the three instruments used in the capsulotomy procedure.

RUPTURES OF THE
ROTATOR CUFF

T HE CONCEPT OF RUPTURES of the musculotendinous cuff or rotator cuff has gained widespread acceptance since the publication of Codman's text, *The Shoulder,* and the subsequent works
of McLaughlin and Moseley. Yet the diagnosis and management
of this entity still remains beclouded with an aura of confusion,
half-truths and misunderstanding. Formerly, the erroneous belief
was prevalent that all patients with a rupture or tear of the cuff
could not abduct the arm well and the "drop-arm test" was positive. The fallacy of this concept could be demonstrated dramati-
cally in acute cases by abolishing the protective pain reflex by the
injection of a local anesthetic agent into the trigger point of tenderness and by observing the patient performing the act of abduction and maintaining this abduction without difficulty. Such patients have only a partial tear or a deep surface tear (Fig. 62).
These types of cases will, as a rule, respond to conservative treatment with the arm placed in a sling for two or three weeks. In
instances where the cuff is torn through its full thickness to expose
the humeral head or is pulled off its attachment from the greater
tuberosity, there is inability to elevate the arm and the patient
may not be able to maintain abduction against the resistance of
the examiner's hand even after an injection of a local anesthetic
around the site of rupture. Patients with complete tears or with
massive ruptures of the cuff (Fig. 63) cannot maintain abduction
at all, and the arm will drop to the side after passive support has
been removed. This so-called "drop-arm sign" is suggestive of a
complete or massive rupture of the rotator cuff. Arthrography is
a very helpful procedure to confirm the clinical findings of a complete tear or even clarify a doubtful diagnosis.

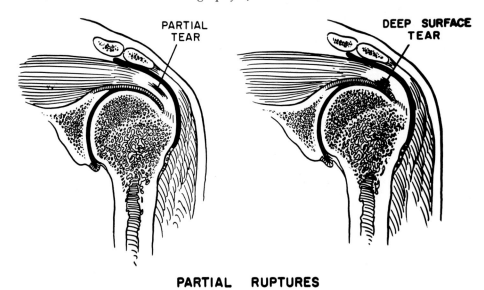

PARTIAL RUPTURES

Figure 62. Usual types of partial ruptures (left) partial tear. (Right) deep surface tear.

In chronic ruptures the diagnosis is much more difficult. These patients are seen primarily for pain in the shoulder but most have good motion, many having 180 degrees of abduction. Their history is that of pain in the shoulder, with or without an injury, of two months' duration or longer. I have seen them treated for periods of six months or more with a diagnosis of frozen shoulder, bursitis or tendinitis because they had a negative "drop-arm test" with good range of shoulder motion or only a slight restriction of motion. If arthrograms had been performed on these patients early, the diagnosis of a rupture could have been made. Exposure of the chronic ruptures at surgery easily explains why these patients have good abduction of the arm. Adhesions are found between the deltoid muscle and the thickened subdeltoid bursa which is also adherent to the rotator cuff, particularly about the site of the rupture. Thus, contraction of the deltoid elevates the arm because of the wide area of fixation of the muscle to the cuff. The tears vary in size from a small rent to a massive tear with retraction of the cuff edges.

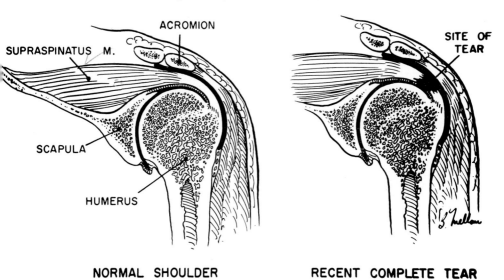

NORMAL SHOULDER   **RECENT COMPLETE TEAR**

Figure 63. Site of rupture at the "critical area" near the insertion of the tendon. (Left) normal shoulder. (Right) recent complete tear.

Tears of one or more components of the rotator cuff occur in one of five ways:

1. There may be a rupture following an injury without a dislocation or a fracture about the shoulder.
2. A rupture may occur following a dislocation of the shoulder.
3. Rupture of the rotator cuff may follow a dislocation of the shoulder with a fracture of the greater tuberosity of the humerus.
4. Chronic Ruptures may occur with or without a history of injury.
5. Tears may occur with avulsion fractures of the greater tuberosity.

RUPTURES OF THE ROTATOR CUFF FOLLOWING AN INJURY WITHOUT A HISTORY OF A DISLOCATION OR FRACTURE

This lesion usually occurs through degenerated tendon tissue. Therefore, it is most frequently seen after the fifth decade of life.

The tendon most commonly ruptured is that of the supraspinatus. Whether the tear is a partial or a complete one, it will generally occur at the "critical area" near the insertion of the tendon into the bony tuberosity of the humerus as seen in Figure 63. This so-called "critical area" is the site where degenerative changes take place, causing a loss of fibrillar structure and elasticity of the tendinous cuff. The patient will usually give a history of a fall, a strain or pushing of the arm, with resulting pain in the shoulder, which is sometimes referred distally to the insertion of the deltoid muscle. There is inability to elevate the arm or hold it in the abducted position. In many instances there may be inability to maintain abduction against resistance of the examiner's hand. If the "drop-arm sign" is positive one may assume that a complete rupture of the cuff is present. If one suspects a parital or incomplete tear, then an injection of a local anesthetic, such as 10 cc of lidocaine, into the suspected area of injury will relieve the protective muscle spasm and accompanying pain. With a partial tear or an incomplete rupture situated in the superficial or deep surface of the cuff or within the substance of the cuff, the patient can usually abduct his arm to about 150 degrees or more. Conservative treatment would then be indicated. With a complete inability to initiate or maintain abduction to at least 90 degrees after the lidocaine injection, arthrography may be performed to confirm the diagnosis of a complete tear. I cannot overemphasize the value of arthrography as a diagnostic aid in complete or massive tears of the rotator cuff of the shoulder.

The appearance of the arthrograms in cases of ruptures will vary as the following cases will demonstrate:

> Arthrograms were done of the right shoulder in a patient forty-nine years of age with the clinical findings of a complete tear of the cuff. The "drop-arm test" was positive. The dye is seen in the subdeltoid bursa with the arm at the side (Fig. 64). With the arm abducted to about 100 degrees, the dependent axillary fold becomes tense; this in turn pushes the dye upward into the subdeltoid bursa and one will observe the bursa further distended with dye (Fig. 65). A complete tear of the cuff was found at operation.

> Arthrograms of the right shoulder of a fifty-three-year-old male barely reveals the outline of the subdeltoid bursa (Fig. 66). Although

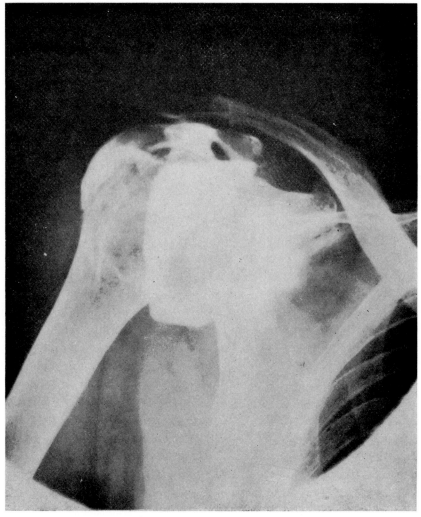

Figure 64. Dye in the subdeltoid bursa indicative of a rupture. Arthrogram taken with the arm at the side.

one can assume that a tear in the cuff exists, an arthrogram taken with the arm abducted to about 90 degrees clearly demonstrates the distended bursa and easily confirms the diagnosis of a rupture (Fig. 67). At operation exposure of the shoulder joint revealed that the patient had a complete rupture of the cuff with some retraction of the cuff edges. The greater tuberosity was bare as the result of the stripping off of its soft tissue components. (Fig. 68).

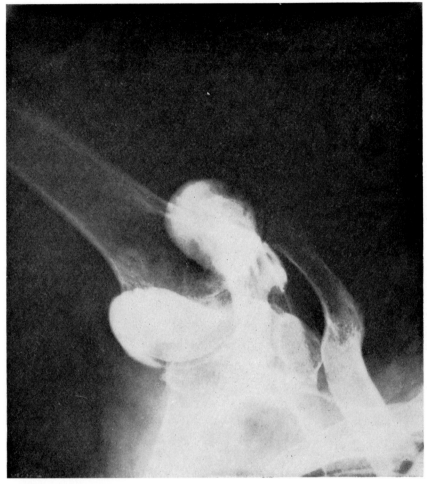

Figure 65. Arthrogram with the arm in some abduction. Dye seen filling the subdeltoid bursa. Convincing evidence of a rupture.

Arthrography was performed on the left shoulder of a fifty-six-year-old male with a suspected tear of the musculotendinous cuff. The films revealed that the dye had extravasated into the subdeltoid bursa (Fig. 69). With the arm in about 110 degrees of abduction the subdeltoid bursa is fully distended with dye (Fig. 70). At operation a complete rupture was found confirming the arthrographic findings.

An unusual arthrographic finding was that of a sixty-one-year-old male who had clinical evidence of a rupture with a positive "drop-arm

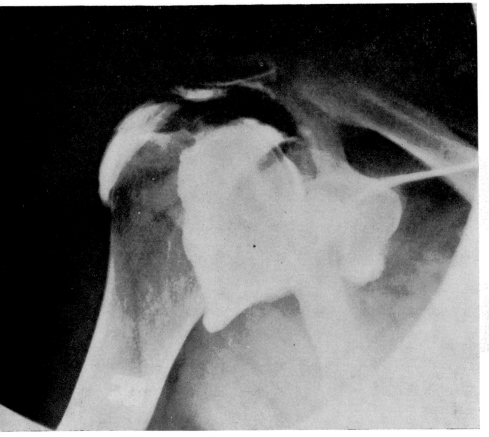

Figure 66. Arthrogram of the right shoulder. The outline of the subdeltoid bursa is barely seen.

test." Note the dye escaping from the subdeltoid bursa into the soft tissues under the deltoid muscle (Fig. 71). At operation this patient had a very large tear of the rotator cuff (Fig. 72).

In another case arthrograms taken of the shoulder in three positions all show evidence of a rupture. Dye is seen in the subdeltoid bursa with the arm by the side in the anterior-posterior view (Fig. 73). With the arm in abduction the "sore thumb" or tongue-like appearance of the bursa is pathognomonic of a rupture (Fig. 74). The axillary view reveals the dye in the bursa which almost forms a circle or halo about the humeral head (Fig. 75). Compare these findings with the normal appearing arthrographic views seen in Figures 18 and 31. An

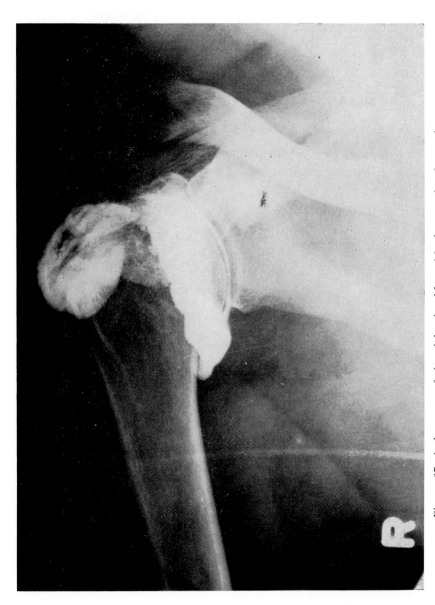

Figure 67. Arthrogram of the right shoulder with the arm in about ninety degrees of abduction. Dye easily fills the subdeltoid bursa to confirm the diagnosis of a rupture.

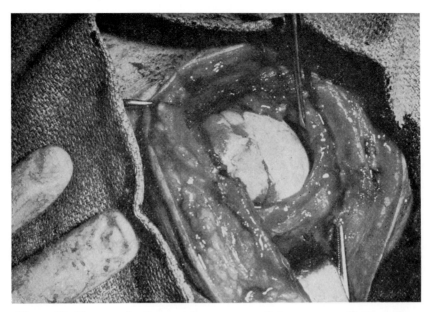

Figure 68. Photograph of a complete rupture of the rotator cuff. Note that the greater tuberosity has been exposed as the result of the stripping off and retraction of its soft tissue components.

arthrogram of another patient with a cuff rupture also shows the circular appearance of the dye about the head of the humerus (Fig. 76).

The arthrograms of a patient, sixty-two years of age, who gave a history of a fall, jerking his right arm and developing a very painful shoulder, were very interesting. On the anterior-posterior view (Fig. 77) most of the dye remained in the bursa superiorly. When the arm was abducted to 90 degrees to obtain an axillary view the dye not only extravasated into the soft tissues posteriorly but also formed a circle about the humeral head because of its presence in the subdeltoid bursa (Fig. 78). At operation the humeral head was completely exposed (Fig. 79) and the greater tuberosity was found to be bare when the ruptured cuff was retracted (Fig. 80).

The treatment of complete tears or massive ruptures is surgical repair. Once the diagnosis is confirmed by arthrography, as evidenced by the extravasation of dye into the subdeltoid bursa, the operation should be performed as soon as possible before the cuff edges are allowed to retract and become scarred or friable.

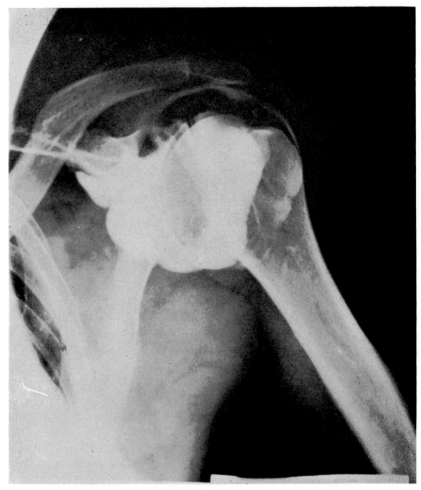

Figure 69. Arthrogram of left shoulder shows some dye in the subdeltoid bursa.

RUPTURE OF THE ROTATOR CUFF FOLLOWING
DISLOCATION OF THE SHOULDER

This is a common injury and a cuff tear may be the only disabling sequela, particularly in the middle-aged or elderly patient. One can easily understand why this is so. When the head of the humerus is pulled out of its normal position, something must give.

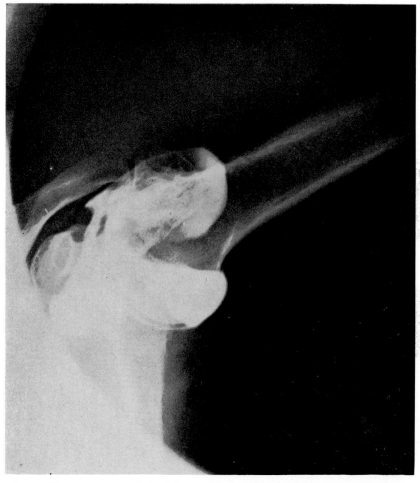

Figure 70. Arthrogram of the left shoulder taken with the left arm abducted to about 110 degrees. Note that the dye has fully distended the subdeltoid bursa. The diagnosis of a rupture was confirmed by operation.

Either the greater tuberosity may fracture or the rotator cuff may tear (Fig. 81). If the X-rays reveal no fracture, one should test the shoulder for a tear. After reduction of the dislocation and immobilization of the arm, the patient can best be tested after an interval of ten to fourteen days. If he does not show any evidence of abduction after the acute phase has subsided, an arthrogram

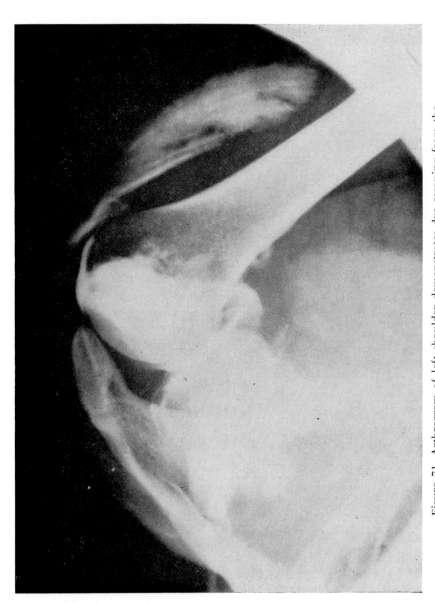

Figure 71. Arthrogram of left shoulder demonstrates dye escaping from the subdeltoid bursa into the soft tissues under the deltoid muscle, also indicative of a rupture.

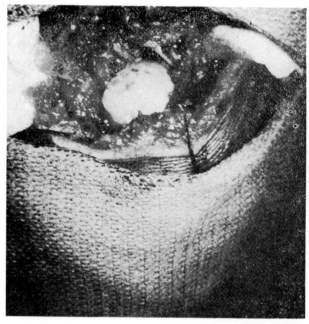

Figure 72. Complete rupture of the rotator cuff. Humeral head completely exposed.

should be considered. This procedure should be done about three weeks following the original injury. An incomplete tear should be healed after this period of time, but a complete or massive rupture should not. If the arthogram reveals evidence of a rupture, then the patient should have the tear repaired. Figure 82 shows the dye being instilled into the joint of a shoulder dislocated twenty-two days previously. The X-ray was taken after 6 cc of dye was injected. No evidence of a rupture was observed on this view. After injection of 16 cc of solution, the dye has filled the subdeltoid bursa with the arm abducted. (Fig. 83). This patient had a complete tear of the rotator cuff. Roentgenographic examinations are most important in the diagnosis of ruptures which follow dislocations. Inasmuch as massive tears are likely to occur in these types of injuries, one should suspect such a lesion subsequent to a reduction if there is an upward riding of the humeral head (Figs. 84 and 85).

Upward displacement of the humeral head is seen in a patient

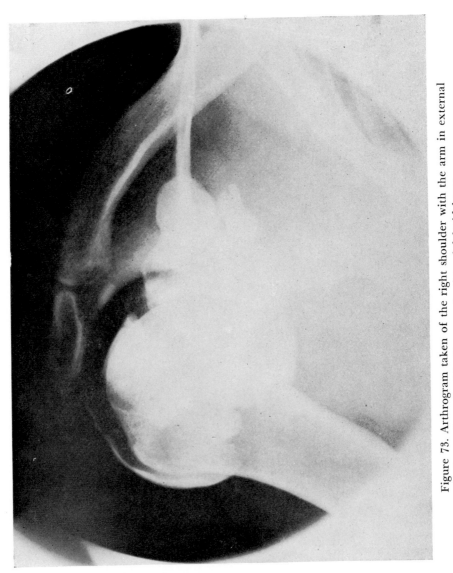

Figure 73. Arthrogram taken of the right shoulder with the arm in external rotation and at the side. Dye seen in the subdeltoid bursa.

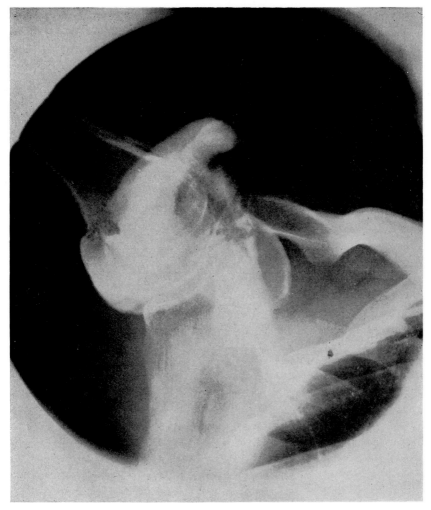

Figure 74. Arthrogram of the right shoulder with the arm in about 110 degrees of abduction. The "sore-thumb" or tongue-like appearance of the dye filled bursa is very definite evidence of an existing rupture.

forty-five years of age who was unable to abduct his arm well one month after reduction of a dislocated shoulder (Fig. 86). The arthrogram is indicative of a rupture, revealing dye in the sub-deltoid bursa (Fig. 87). At operation a massive irregular tear was found (Fig. 88). Note the exposure of the head of the humerus

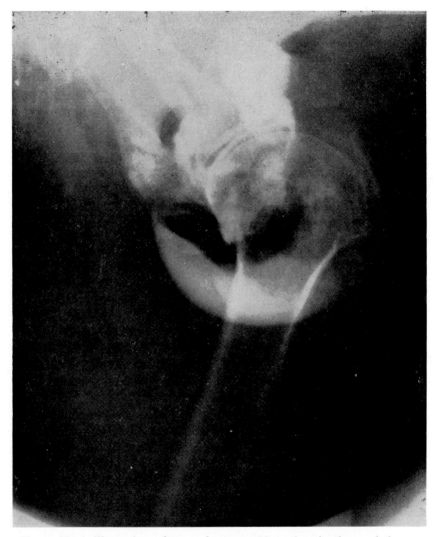

Figure 75. Axillary view of an arthrogram. Note the circular or halo appearance of the dye filled bursa about the humeral head. Another indication of a rupture.

and the hook about the biceps tendon. This upward riding of the humeral head is due to lack of support of the overlaying structures as the tear extended through the full thickness of the tendons, joint capsule and possibly the floor of the bursa. Since the force of

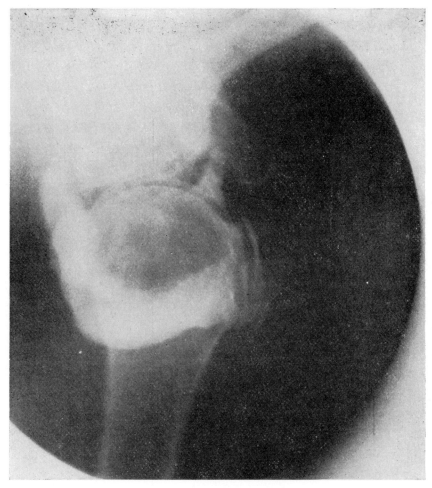

Figure 76. Axillary view of an arthrogram showing circular appearance of dye in the subdeltoid bursa indicative of a rupture.

the short rotators is lost, the deltoid acting alone elicits an upward force resulting in an upward displacement or subluxation of the humeral head. With the patient standing, an inferior subluxation of the head of the humerus may be demonstrated by roentgenograms taken with the arm hanging down or holding a heavy weight. In addition, there are certain instances of dislocations when, after reduction, a persistent downward subluxation of the humeral head may occur; if this is so, it generally indicates a large

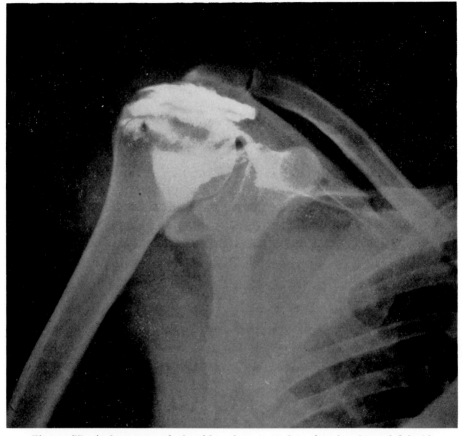

Figure 77. Arthrogram of shoulder demonstrating dye in the subdeltoid bursa suggestive of a rupture. (Courtesy of *A.A.O.S. Instructional Course Lectures, 13*:209, 1956.)

cuff tear. This is usually seen in elderly patients where the degenerative changes in the rotator cuff are most pronounced. The weight of the arm acts as a downward force. If there should be either an upward riding or a subluxation inferiorly of the head of the humerus and the patient has a definite disability, he should have the tear repaired after the arthrograms have confirmed the clinical findings.

The approaches to the shoulder for the repair of small tears or fresh ruptures of the rotator cuff are the acromioclavicular arthro-

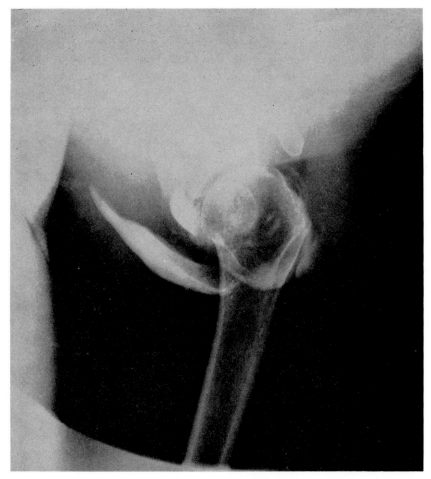

Figure 78. Axillary view of arthrogram of patient shown in Figure 77. Note circular appearance of the dye in the subdeltoid bursa as well as some dye extravasating into the soft tissues posteriorly. (Courtesy of *A.A.O.S. Instructional Course Lectures, 13*:209, 1956.)

plasty described by Bateman, the anterior acromioplasty described by Neer or the transacromial approach using the sabre cut incision. I have found the latter approach the most desirable one for repairing massive tears and ideal for the repair of chronic ruptures.

All cuff tears should be repaired without tension; if this is not

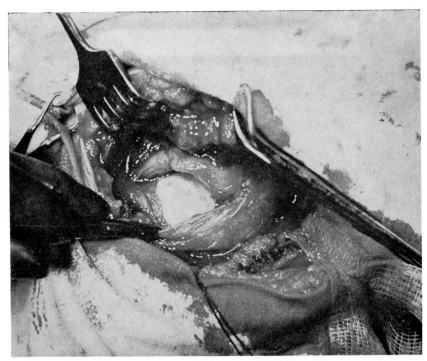

Figure 79. Humeral head exposed through the ruptured rotator cuff. (Courtesy of *A.A.O.S. Instructional Course Lectures, 13*:209, 1956.)

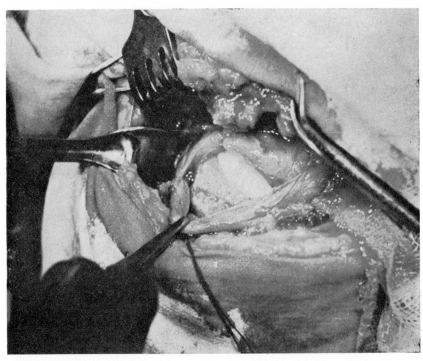

Figure 80. Torn cuff retracted exposing the greater tuberosity which is bare. (Courtesy of *A.A.O.S. Instructional Course Lectures, 13*:209, 1956.)

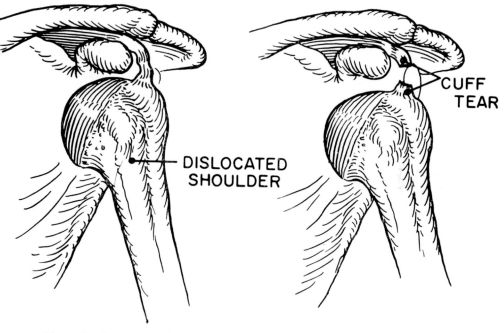

DISLOCATED SHOULDER

CUFF TEAR

Figure 81. In a dislocation of the shoulder the cuff may tear.

possible one may use the biceps tendon as a free graft or a freeze-dried rotator cuff. This will be discussed under "Chronic Ruptures." Rarely is it necessary to suture the cuff medially in a groove in the head of the humerus (Fig. 89) or fuse the shoulder joint (Fig. 90) .

RUPTURE OF THE ROTATOR CUFF FOLLOWING DISLOCATION OF THE SHOULDER WITH A FRACTURE OF THE GREATER TUBEROSITY OF THE HUMERUS

Dislocation of the shoulder with a fracture of the greater tuberosity nearly always is accompanied by a torn cuff in some form. Although this may be our most frequent injury, as far as cuff tears are concerned, many such tears do not require operative repair. This is particularly true if the tuberosity fragment falls into its normal position after the dislocation is reduced. However, some of these cases may result in serious disability if they are not managed properly. The roentgenograms will provide a clue regarding

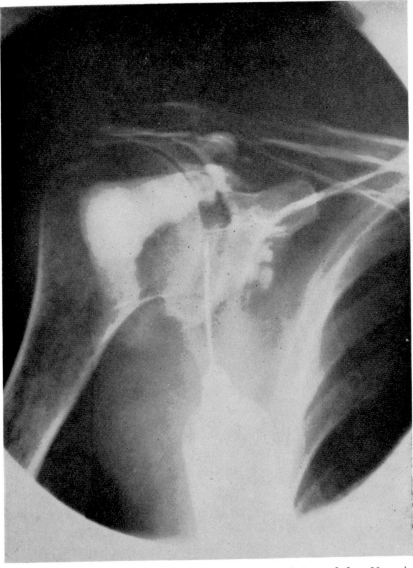

Figure 82. Roentgenogram taken after instillation of 6 cc of dye. No evidence of rupture seen at this time.

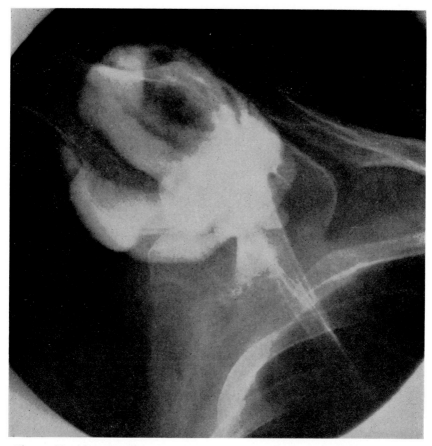

Figure 83. After instillation of 16 cc of dye and the arm placed in some abduction the subdeltoid bursa is well-outlined indicating the presence of a ruptured rotator cuff.

the necessity for operative intervention. The greater tuberosity fragment will assume one of three positions (Fig. 91). It will remain in its normal position opposite the glenoid, it may be retracted under the acromion, or it may follow the humeral head.

If the greater tuberosity fragment remains in its normal position opposite the glenoid (Fig. 92) there is generally a tear of the aponeurosis between the lesser and greater tuberosities, allowing the humeral head to dislocate. This dislocation is usually intracapsular. When the dislocation is reduced, the tuberosity fragment

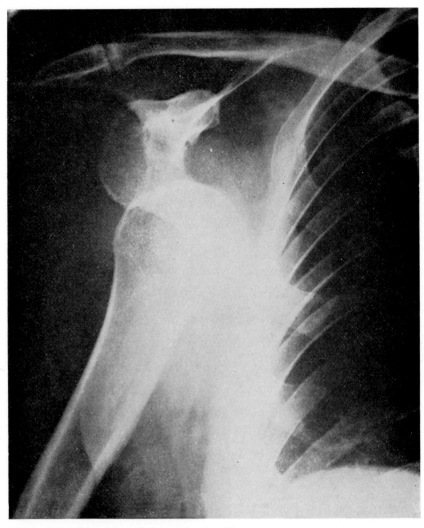

Figure 84. Dislocation of the right shoulder.

falls into its normal position and the edges of the longitudinal tear heal well with good function (Fig. 93). Even if the greater tuberosity should follow the head (Fig. 94), after reduction the fragment may assume its normal position (Fig. 95). Fortunately, this is the most common occurrence in fracture dislocation of the shoulder. One should never reduce the dislocation and immo-

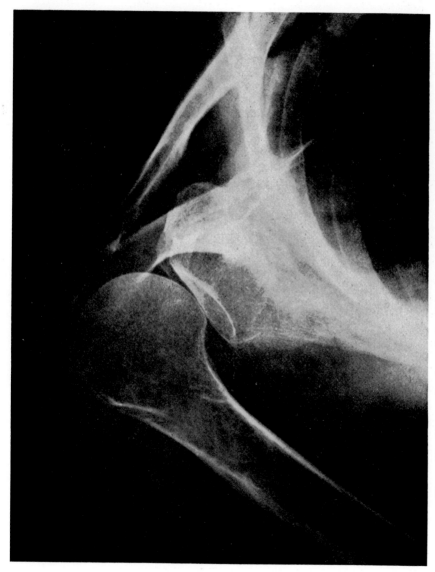

Figure 85. After reduction of the dislocation. Upward riding of the head of the humerus in relation to the glenoid.

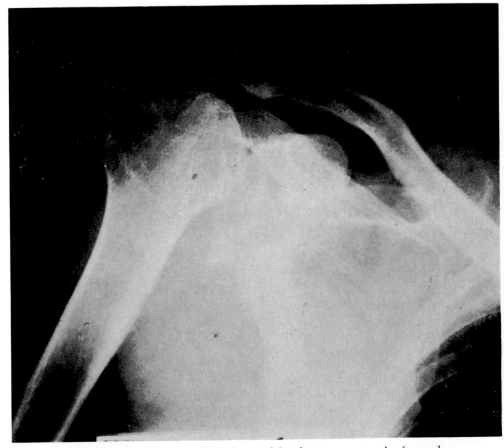

Figure 86. Upward riding of the humeral head seen one month after reduction of a dislocated shoulder.

bilize the arm in abduction with the hope of maintaining the fragment in its normal position. The tuberosity fragment will abut against the acromial arch and will remain displaced (Fig. 96). It may fall into a normal position with the arm at the side as shown in Figure 93. It should be emphasized that the physiological position is with the arm at the side and not in the abducted position.

There are instances in a dislocation when the tuberosity fragment will either follow the head or remain opposite the glenoid, yet will not return to its normal position after the shoulder has been reduced. Then the treatment becomes a surgical problem.

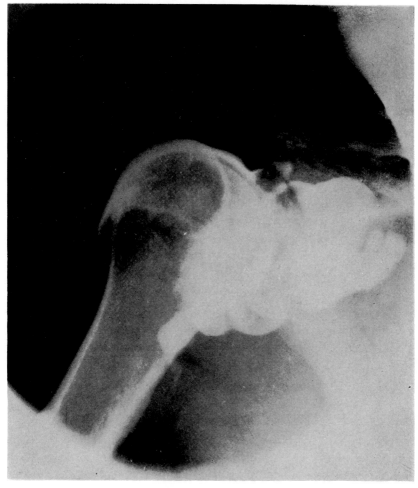

Figure 87. Arthrogram reveals dye in the subdeltoid bursa confirming clinical evidence of a rupture.

Since the three external rotators of the shoulder are attached to the greater tuberosity, this fragment must be placed in a satisfactory position if one hopes to obtain a good functioning shoulder. The following cases illustrate the problems:

A sixty-six-year-old male fell and dislocated his left shoulder. In addition to the dislocation he had a fracture of the greater tuberosity (Fig. 97). After reduction of the dislocation the greater tuberosity

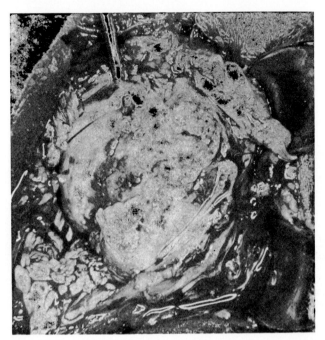

Figure 88. Massive irregular tear seen following a dislocation which had been reduced one month previously. Note hook about the exposed biceps tendon.

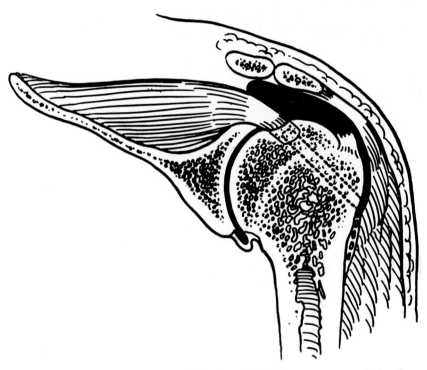

Figure 89. Edges of the torn cuff fixed medially in a groove made in the head of the humerus.

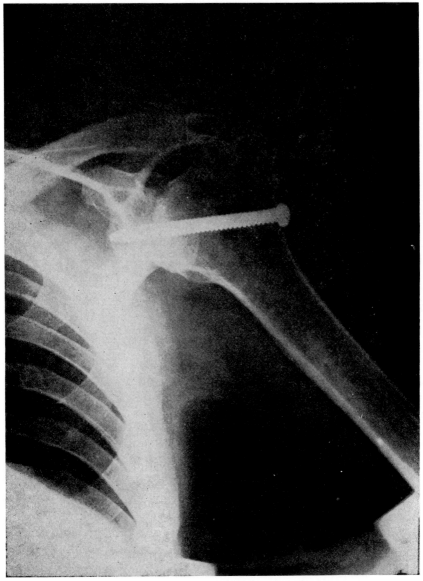

Figure 90. Shoulder fused after removing the articular cartilage from the glenoid and humeral head and using a screw for internal fixation.

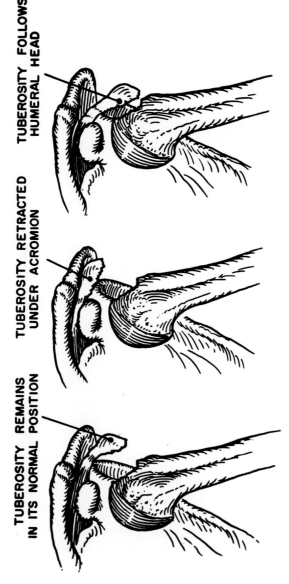

Figure 91. In a dislocation of the shoulder with a fracture of the greater tuberosity, the tuberosity fragment will assume one of three positions.

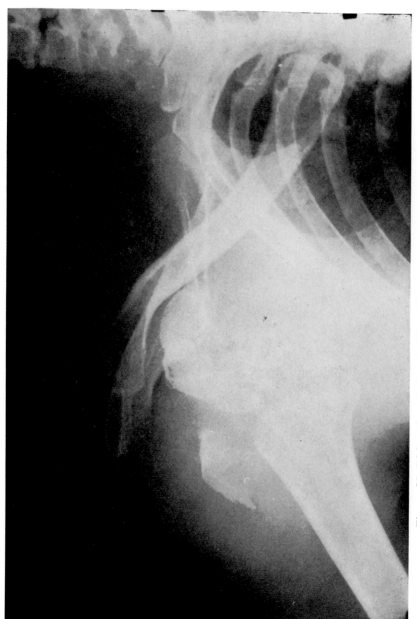

Figure 92. Dislocation of the shoulder with the greater tuberosity fragment remaining opposite the glenoid. (Courtesy of *J. Bone Joint Surgery, 44-A:* 984, July, 1962.)

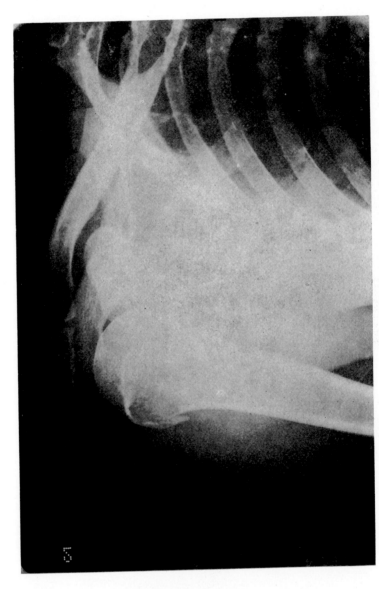

Figure 93. After reduction of the dislocation the tuberosity fragment falls into a satisfactory position. (Courtesy of *J. Bone Joint Surgery, 44-A:984,* July, 1962.)

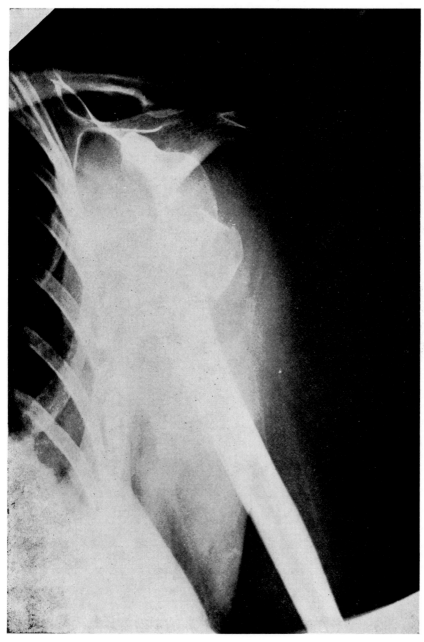

Figure 94. Greater tuberosity has followed the head when dislocated.

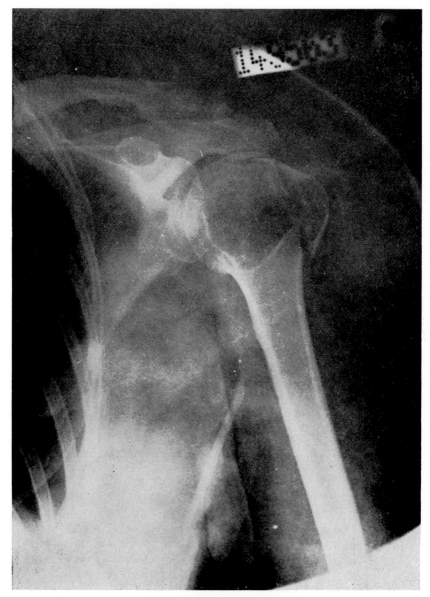

Figure 95. The greater tuberosity fragment assumes a relatively normal position after reduction of the dislocation.

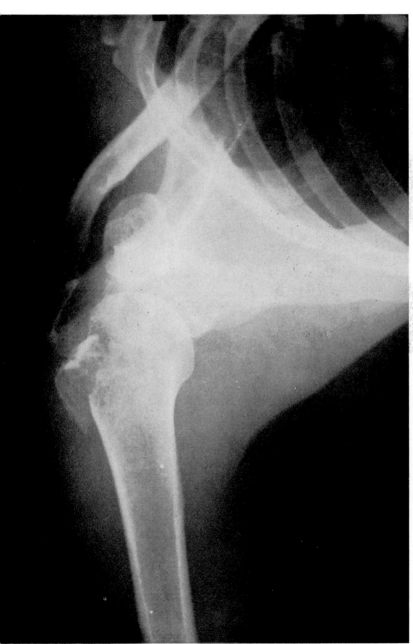

Figure 96. The dislocation of the shoulder seen in Figure 92 has been reduced and the arm placed in abduction. Note the unsatisfactory position of the greater tuberosity. (Courtesy of *J. Bone Joint Surgery, 44-A:984,* July, 1962.)

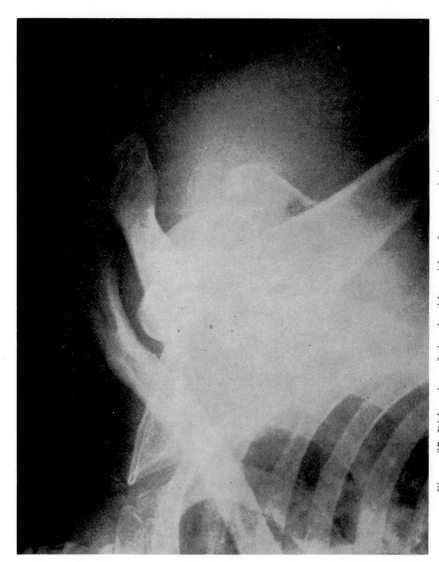

Figure 97. Dislocation of the shoulder with a fracture of the greater tuberosity. The fragment has followed the head. (Courtesy of *A.A.O.S. Instructional Course Lectures, 13:212,* 1956.)

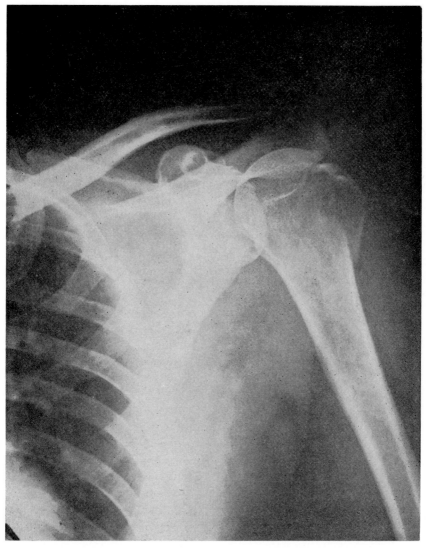

Figure 98. After reduction of the dislocation the tuberosity fragment remains displaced laterally and somewhat downward. (Courtesy of *A.A.O.S. Instructional Course Lectures, 13:*213, 1956.)

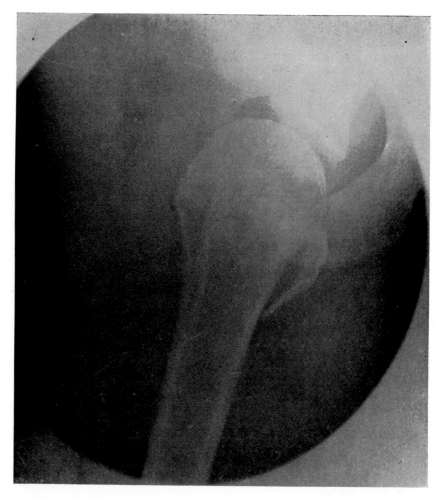

Figure 99. Axillary view reveals the greater tuberosity fragment to be retracted posteriorly. (Courtesy of *A.A.O.S. Instructional Course Lectures, 13*:213, 1956.)

fragment remained displaced laterally as well as downward (Fig. 98) and retracted posteriorly as seen on the axillary view (Fig. 99). Even with the arm placed in some abduction the tuberosity fragment still remained displaced (Fig. 100). At operation a large bony defect was seen adjacent to the head of the humerus (Fig. 101). This is not an unusual finding in a case with a displaced greater tuberosity fragment.

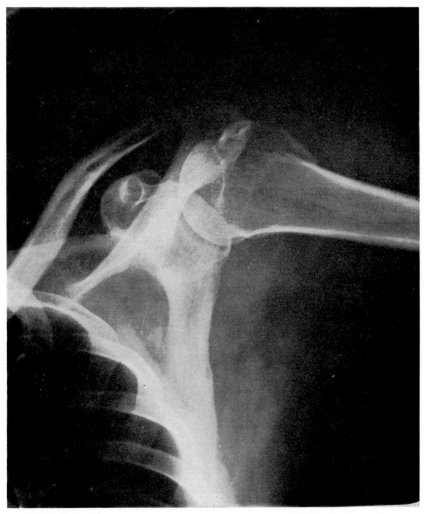

Figure 100. With arm in some abduction the tuberosity is still displaced downward. (Courtesy of *A.A.O.S. Instructional Course Lectures, 13:213,* 1956.)

The following case demonstrates how the rotator cuff is torn about the edges of the greater tuberosity when it is fractured and displaced.

This fifty-six-year-old male dislocated his left shoulder. After reduction the greater tuberosity fragment remained displaced (Fig. 102)

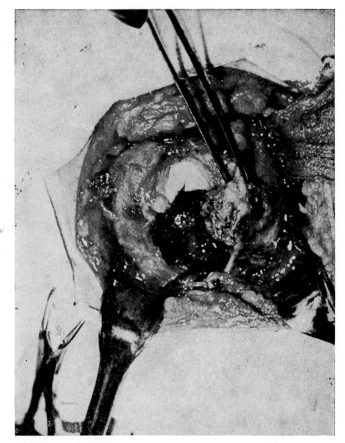

Figure 101. The tuberosity fragment is held by a forceps. Notice the large bony defect adjacent to the humeral head. (Courtesy of *A.A.O.S. Instructional Course Lectures, 13:*213, 1956.)

and on the axillary view it is seen posteriorly (Fig. 103). The arthrograms show the dye escaping around the fracture site due to the tear of the cuff edges about the tuberosity (Fig. 104). The axillary view reveals the fragment still retracted posteriorly with some dye escaping from its superior posterior edges (Fig. 105).

The following cases demonstrate how this problem can be solved:

A forty-four-year-old male sustained a fracture-dislocation of the left shoulder (Fig. 106). The tuberosity fragment remained opposite the

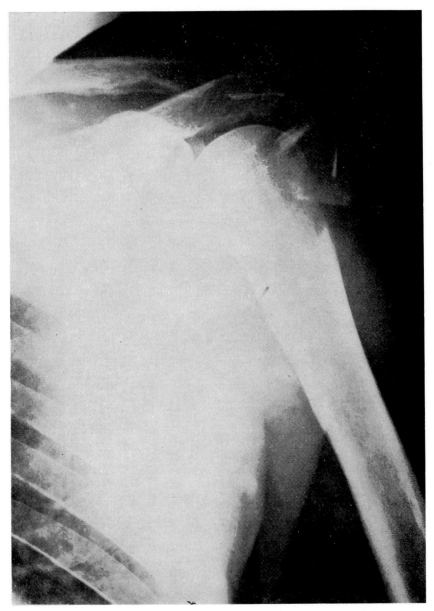

Figure 102. The greater tuberosity fragment remains displaced after reduction of a dislocation.

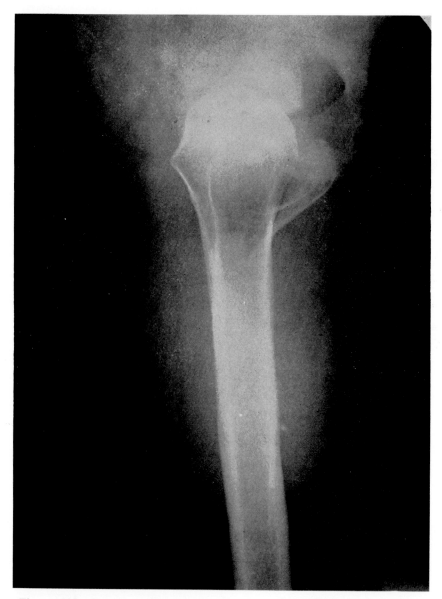

Figure 103. On the axillary view the tuberosity fragment is displaced posteriorly.

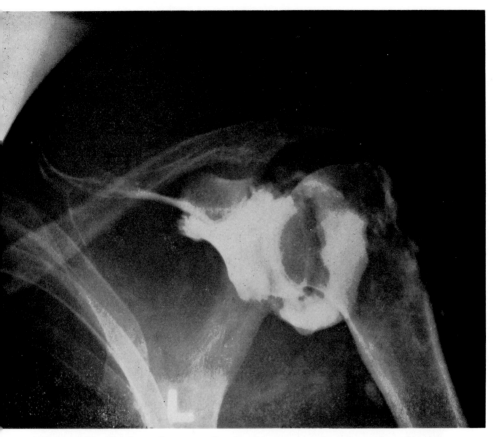

Figure 104. On the arthrogram the dye is seen escaping about the edges of the cuff at the site of the fractured tuberosity fragment.

glenoid when the head was dislocated but did not resume its normal position after reduction of the dislocation (Fig. 107). The axillary view revealed the tuberosity fragment displaced posteriorly by the pull of the external rotators (Fig. 108). Since the function of the external rotators would be poor or useless in this position, operative reduction was performed through the superior approach and the fragment fixed in its normal position by two screws (Fig. 109). The cuff edges were sutured together after the fragment had been fixed secured in position by the screws.

In another instance, if the tuberosity fragment should follow the humeral head at the time of the dislocation (Fig. 110) one

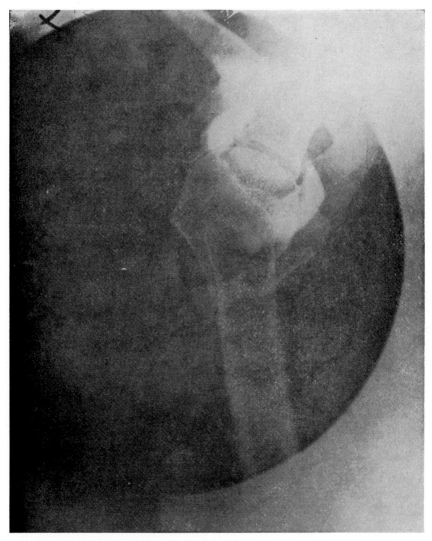

Figure 105. On the axillary view the dye is seen escaping superiorly and posteriorly about the fracture site.

should be very suspicious of a cuff tear. This is particularly true, if, after reduction of the dislocation the tuberosity fragment is not restored to its normal position (Figs. 111, 112). Surgical reduction of the fracture becomes necessary to place the fragment in its original position (Figs. 113, 114).

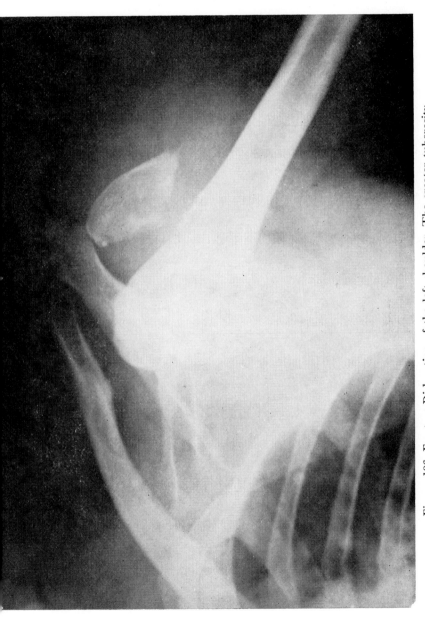

Figure 106. Fracture-Dislocation of the left shoulder. The greater tuberosity fragment remains opposite the glenoid. (Courtesy of *A.A.O.S. Instructional Course Lectures*, 13:212, 1956.)

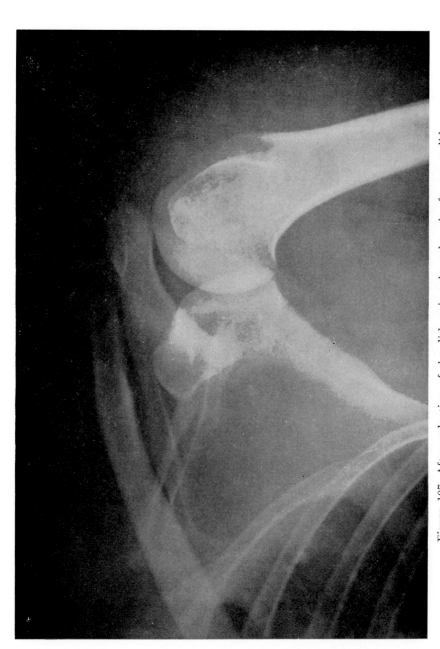

Figure 107. After reduction of the dislocation the tuberosity fragment did not resume its normal position. (Courtesy of *A.A.O.S. Instructional Course Lectures, 13:212,* 1956.)

Figure 108. The axillary view reveals the tuberosity fragment displaced posteriorly. (Courtesy of *A.A.O.S. Instructional Course Lectures, 13*:212, 1956.)

It may be difficult for one to realize the extent of the tear that does exist when the greater tuberosity fragment has been fractured off its attachment from the humerus. Only at operation can this be seen. When the fragment is replaced, fixed with a screw and the edges of the cuff sutured (Figs. 115, 116), then one may anticipate a satisfactorily functioning shoulder. Figure 117 shows a case where only a single screw was used to fix the tuberosity fragment

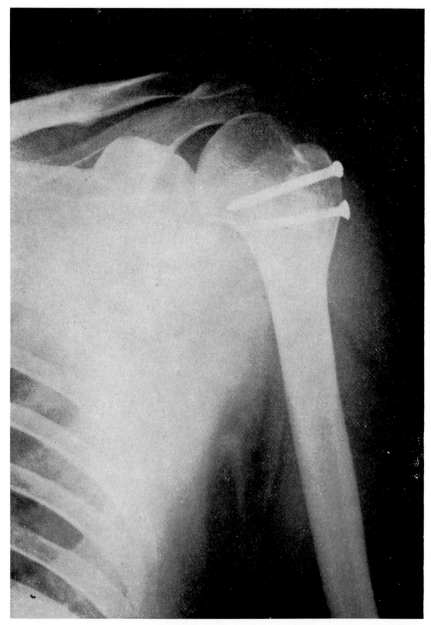

Figure 109. After open reduction the greater tuberosity fragment is now restored to its normal position and fixed by two screws. (Courtesy of *A.A.O.S. Instructional Course Lectures, 13*:212, 1956.)

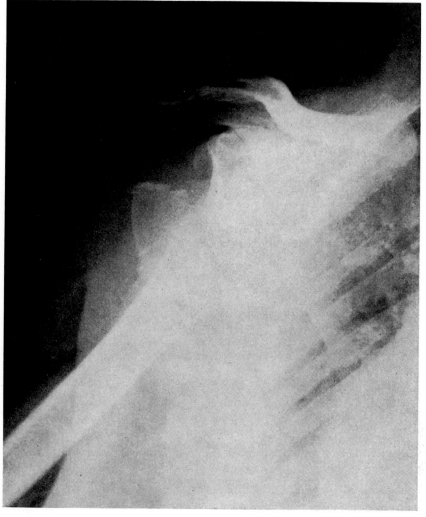

Figure 110. Fracture-dislocation of the shoulder. The tuberosity fragment follows the head.

in position. This is possible occasionally when the fragment is in one piece and not comminuted.

If the tuberosity fragment should be retracted up under the acromion after reduction of the dislocation (Figs. 118, 119), one must presume a large and extensive tear exists. In addition, the

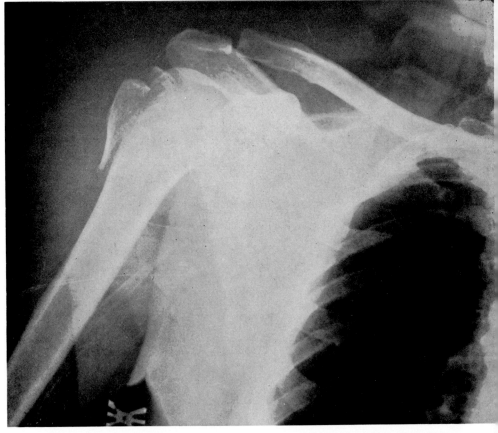

Figure 111. After reduction the tuberosity is not in good position. It is held in external rotation and also displaced downward and posteriorly.

tuberosity fragment under the acromion acts as a wedge between the humerus and the acromion restricting glenohumeral motion and blocking full abduction. The pull or leverage of the external rotators is also lost because of the foreshortened distance of the muscles. Since the function of the shoulder is impaired it is mandatory that such a patient be operated upon and the fragment replaced. Early operative repair should be done through the transacromial approach with restoration of the tuberosity fragment to the shaft of the humerus by sutures or screws. I prefer the screw, as this allows the patient to start early motion, resulting in a

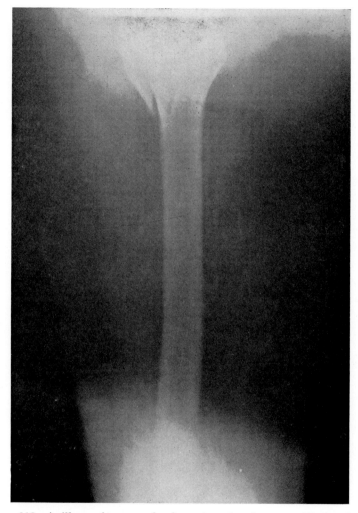

Figure 112. Axillary view reveals the tuberosity fragment displaced posteriorly.

shorter postoperative period of disability. There can be instances where the fragment is quite comminuted and impossible to replace securely. If this is so, then the fragment should be excised and discarded, the cuff fixed to the humerus by screws (Figs. 120, 121), and the edges sutured to that part of the cuff remaining at the periphery of the fracture site.

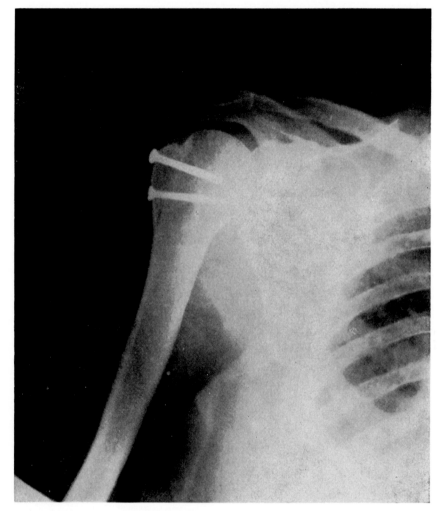

Figure 113. After operation the greater tuberosity is held in excellent position by two screws.

CHRONIC RUPTURES OF THE MUSCULOTENDINOUS CUFF WITH OR WITHOUT A HISTORY OF AN INJURY

This lesion appears to be poorly understood and frequently it is overlooked or missed altogether. This is due to two common misconceptions propounded by many authors in the past. These impressions concerning ruptures of the rotator cuff are that rup-

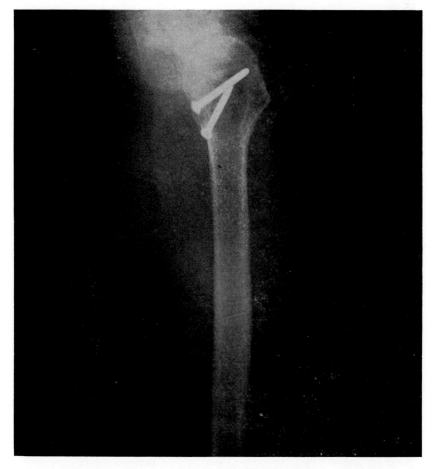

Figure 114. Axillary view also shows the tuberosity fixed in good position.

tures are rather infrequent, and that patients with ruptures have limited motion, cannot elevate the involved arm well and have a positive "drop-arm test". Neither of these is true, particularly in cases of chronic ruptures where the main complaint is that of pain which has been present for two months or more. In such cases the clinical findings can be misleading since there is generally a good range of abduction present. If there is any doubt as to the diagnosis, the patient should undergo arthrography. It will confirm the diagnosis of a tear. Surgery is then indicated for repair of the rup-

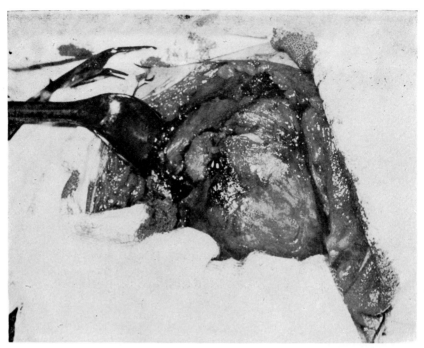

Figure 115. Tuberosity fragment seen in Figure 101 is fixed in position by a screw.

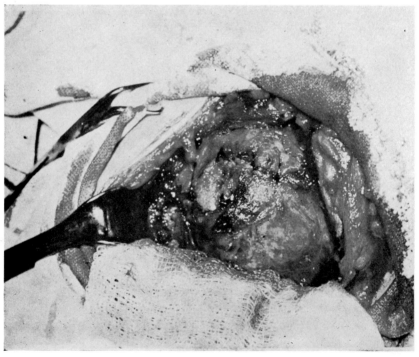

Figure 116. After insertion of the screw the cuff edges are sutured.

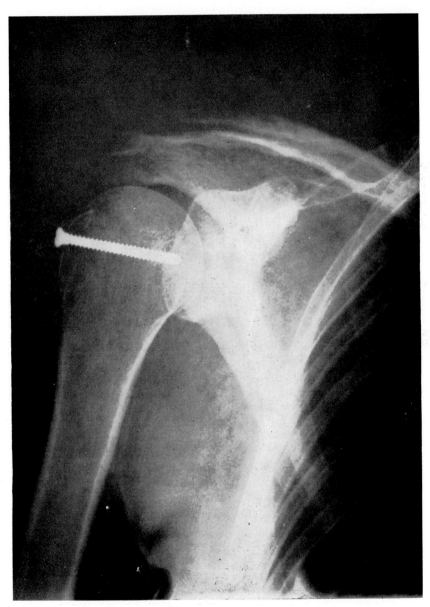

Figure 117. Greater tuberosity fragment is fixed in satisfactory position with only one screw.

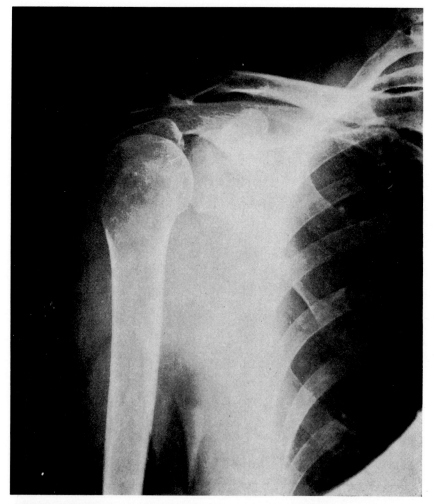

Figure 118. After reduction of the dislocation the greater tuberosity is retracted under the acromion. (Courtesy of *A.A.O.S. Instructional Lectures, 13:212,* 1956.)

ture, and, if necessary, the long head of the biceps tendon can be used as a free graft to close the shoulder capsule.

The following cases will illustrate the points emphasized:

A fifty-nine-year-old male was seen seven months following a fall off a ladder. He had sustained a dislocation of his right shoulder. After

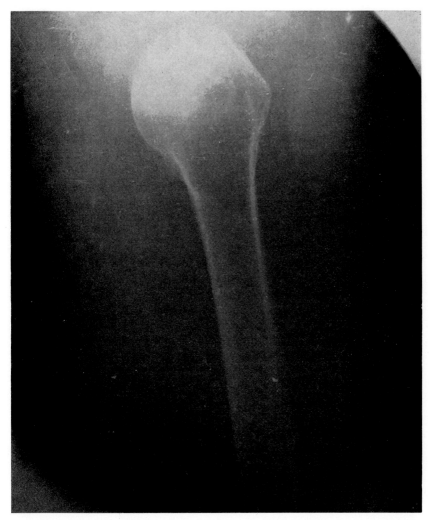

Figure 119. Axillary view reveals a large space just below the anatomical neck where the tuberosity fragment has been pulled away from its normal site.

reduction of the dislocation the arm was immobilized for three weeks. Following this he was given physical therapy and exercises. When his pain and limitation of motion continued a manipulation of his shoulder was performed under general anesthesia for a frozen shoulder. This procedure, done about two months after his injury, gave him no relief. Another manipulation was performed two weeks later. Physical

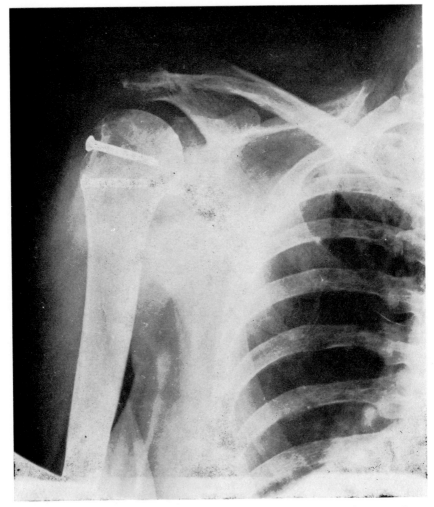

Figure 120. After open reduction the comminuted tuberosity fragment has been discarded and the cuff fixed in its former position by two screws. (Courtesy of *A.A.O.S. Instructional Lectures*, *13*:212, 1956.)

therapy was again instituted but when his pain continued, a third manipulation under general anesthesia was performed two months after the second manipulation. When the patient's symptoms were not relieved the orthopedic surgeon referred him to me. Although active abduction was 150 degrees his main complaint was pain. An arthrogram revealed evidence of a rupture (Fig. 122). At operation, per-

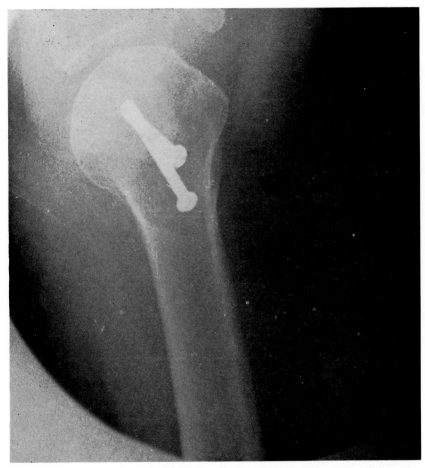

Figure 121. Axillary view. Cuff fixed just below the anatomical neck by two screws.

formed nine months after his injury, a large irregular tear was found (Fig. 123). Since the edges of the cuff could not be approximated a free biceps tendon graft was used to cover the defect in the cuff (Fig. 124). The patient did quite well and he returned to work as a bus driver two months after his operation or eleven months after his injury. When last examined about one year after his operation he had minimal discomfort. Active abduction was 170 degrees and upon internal rotation he was able to reach seven inches above the belt line.

A forty-one-year-old male was seen about two and one-half months after his injury. While pushing a large piece of plywood board he felt

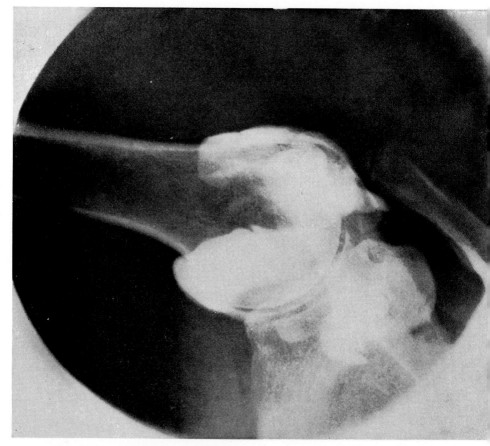

Figure 122. Arthrogram of the right shoulder taken with the arm at ninety degrees of abduction. Dye is forced superiorly into the subdeltoid bursa indicative of a rupture.

pain in his right shoulder. He was seen by an orthopedic surgeon and was given medication for pain. No other therapy was prescribed. His pain continued until he reached the point he could not sleep. Active abduction was 135 degrees. An arthrogram performed four days later revealed extravasation of dye into the subdeltoid bursa. Surgery was performed five weeks later through the superior approach. A large tear of the rotator cuff was noted. When the cuff edges could not be approximated the biceps tendon was resected proximally (Fig. 125) and used as a free graft after sectioning it in a book-like manner (Fig. 126). Examination eighteen months later revealed active abduction to

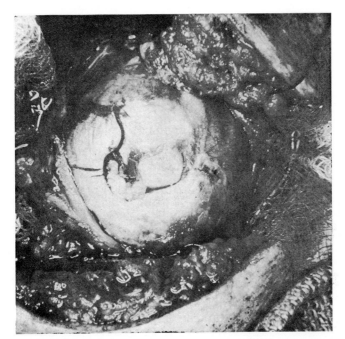

Figure 123. A large irregular cuff tear with retraction of the cuff edges seen nine months after injury.

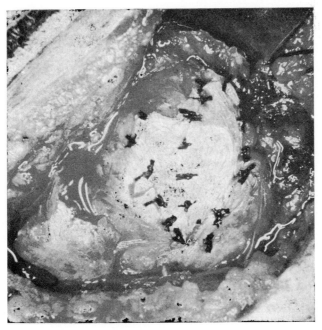

Figure 124. A free biceps graft easily covers the defect in the cuff.

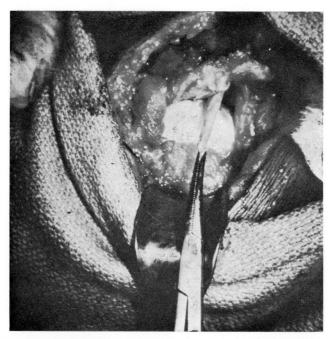

Figure 125. The long head of the biceps has been resected proximally prior to being used as a free graft.

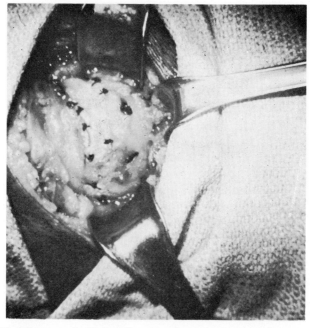

Figure 126. The capsule is closed using the biceps tendon as a free graft.

170 degrees. His pain had subsided and the patient was able to sleep without any medication.

A forty-six-year-old male was first seen two and one-half months after an injury complaining of pain in his right shoulder radiating down the right arm. He stated that he was working on some valves and felt something pull in his shoulder. He was seen by an orthopedist and was given physical therapy without relief. When it was suggested that he have a resection of the outer third of the clavicle, the patient was referred to me. Active abduction was 145 degrees with no points of tenderness elicited about the shoulder joint. An arthrogram performed four days later revealed dye in the subdeltoid bursa, indicating a rupture (Figs. 127, 128). Surgery was performed two weeks later and,

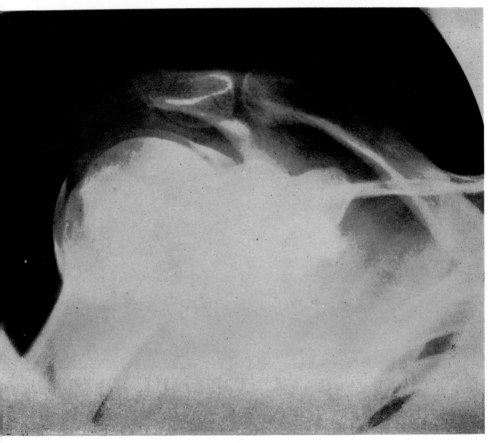

Figure 127. Arthrogram reveals dye in the subdeltoid bursa.

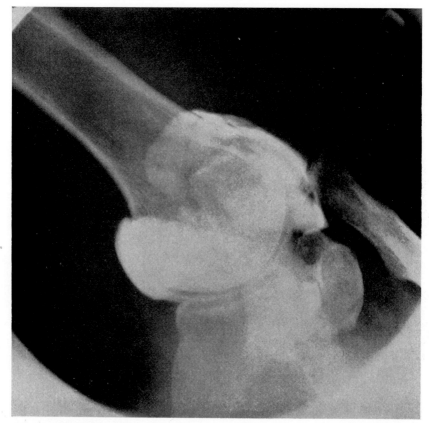

Figure 128. With the arm in some abduction the dye completely fills the subdeltoid bursa.

upon exposure of the joint, it was noted that the subscapularis tendon was torn from the lesser tuberosity anteriorly. In addition, the external rotator tendons were retracted. It was impossible to bring the cuff edges together (Fig. 129) so a free biceps tendon graft was used placing the glistening surface towards the humeral head. In this manner we were able to close the gap in the rotator cuff (Fig. 130). This patient did well postoperatively. He was relieved of most of his pain and when last seen three years later he could abduct to 175 degrees (Fig. 131).

A male patient, sixty-six years of age, had been complaining of pain in the right shoulder for a period of about four months. The patient could not recall any definite history of an injury. Active abduction

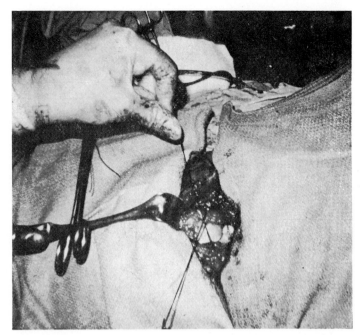

Figure 129. Observe the gap in the cuff even with the sutures being pulled under tension.

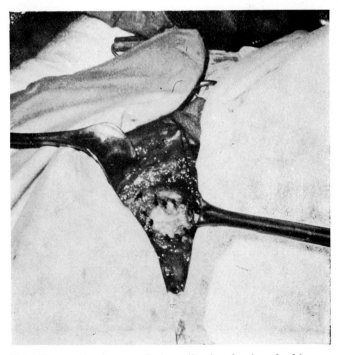

Figure 130. The gap in the capsule is easily closed using the biceps as a free graft.

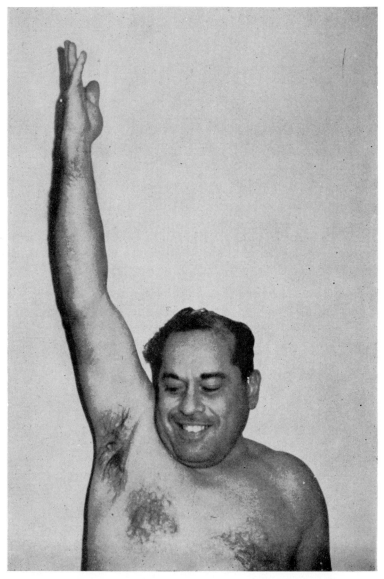

Figure 131. Patient could abduct to 175 degrees when last seen two and one half years after operation. Pain was minimal.

was 175 degrees. An arthrogram revealed dye in the subdeltoid bursa. At operation a large irregular tear was found (Fig. 132). After excising the ragged edges the cuff could not be sutured end to end or side to side. A free biceps graft was used to close the gap in the capsule (Fig. 133). A follow-up twenty-one months later revealed 160 degrees of active abduction. The patient was able to use his arm with very little discomfort.

A forty-two-year-old male was seen six months after an injury. He stated he was discharging a passenger from his car when another vehicle ran into the rear of his car. He complained of pain in his neck and right shoulder. When he was taken to the hospital his cervical spine was X-rayed and the patient was given a collar to wear. The shoulder was treated with suprascapular blocks, and subsequently, when he did not improve, instillations of a refined steroid and lidocaine were given into the capsule. Originally, active abduction was 180 degrees and the other motions of the right shoulder were within normal limits. At the time of my examination active abduction was 100 degrees and passive abduction was 160 degrees. The patient's main complaints were pain and stiffness in the shoulder. An arthrogram performed on the right shoulder revealed dye in the subdeltoid bursa (Figs. 134, 135). A large tear was found at operation, and the humeral head was easily seen through the ruptured cuff (Fig. 136). The gap in the cuff could not be closed without tension, so a free biceps graft was used to cover the head (Fig. 137). Following operative repair of the torn rotator cuff, the patient slowly regained much of his motion and when seen four months after operation active and passive abduction were 170 degrees. He returned to work as a chauffeur nine weeks after operation.

A fifty-five-year-old male slipped on some grease on the floor, falling with his right arm outstretched. He developed pain in his shoulder. He was treated with physical therapy and medication. When seen by me three months later he could abduct his shoulder to 160 degrees. Arthrography confirmed the suspected diagnosis of a rupture. At operation a large irregular tear was noted (Fig. 138). Upon closer observation the biceps tendon can be seen overlying the humeral head. The defect in the cuff was closed readily with a free biceps graft when the cuff edges could not be approximated without tension (Fig. 139).

Technique for Repair of a Ruptured Rotator Cuff using the Biceps Tendon as a Free Graft

The usual approach is the sabre cut incision with the patient in the sitting position and the arm draped free (Fig. 140). After osteotomizing the outer portion of the acromion the deltoid is re-

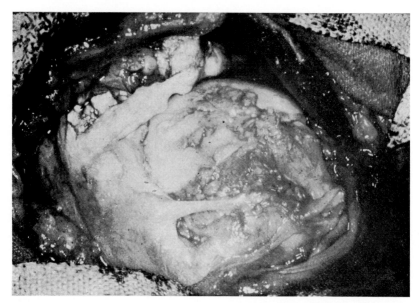

Figure 132. Note the markedly irregular cuff edges found four months after an injury.

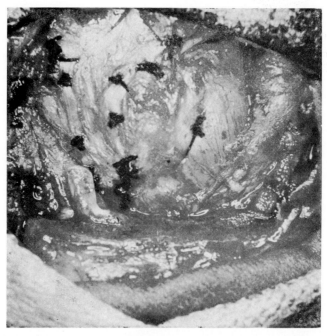

Figure 133. After excising the irregular cuff edges the capsule is closed using the biceps tendon as a free graft.

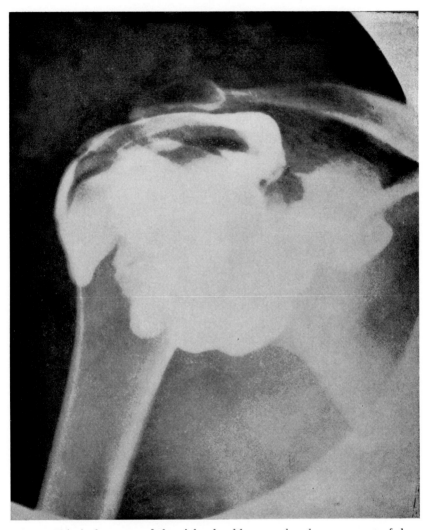

Figure 134. Arthrogram of the right shoulder reveals a large amount of dye present in the subdeltoid confirming a suspected diagnosis of a rupture of the rotator cuff.

tracted downward. If necessary, the deltoid may be stripped from the lateral portion of the clavicle to get better exposure. Adhesions between the subdeltoid bursa and under the surface of the deltoid are separated by the use of the fingers or a wide periosteal elevator. Once this has been accomplished the thickened bursa is opened.

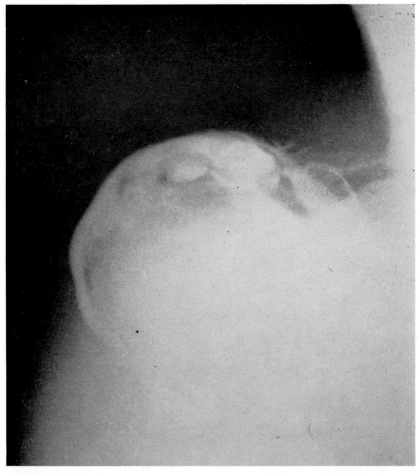

Figure 135. Bicipital groove view of an arthrogram. Note the circular appearance of the dye around the humeral head. The biceps sheath is well outlined in the bicipital groove.

Adhesions between the bursa and rotator cuff are also separated. Once this is done the full extent of the tear or rupture can be easily visualized (Fig. 141). When the edges of the cuff cannot be sutured side to side or end to end without tension then a free biceps graft is used. The intraarticular portion of the biceps is sectioned close to its attachment to the supraglenoid tuberosity and cut distally at the level of the upper part of the bicipital

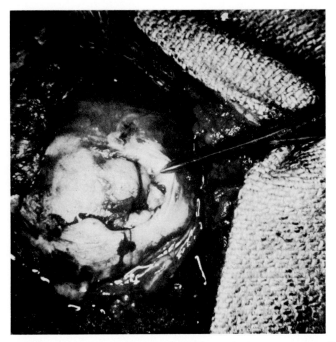

Figure 136. Humeral head easily visualized through the ruptured cuff edges. (Courtesy *Arch Surgery, 102:*483–485, May, 1971, Copyright 1971, AMA).

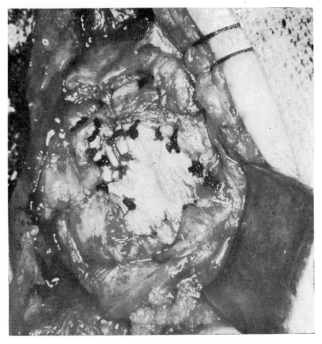

Figure 137. The biceps graft easily closes the capsular defect without tension.

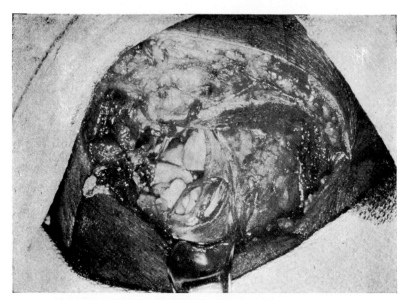

Figure 138. Rupture of rotator cuff. Observe the biceps tendon overlying the humeral head.

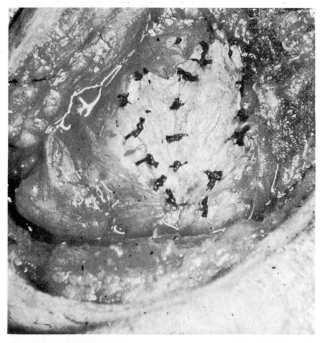

Figure 139. Defect in the cuff closed without tension using a free biceps graft.

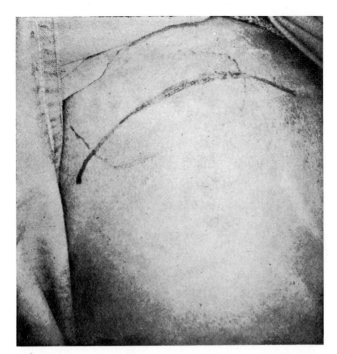

Figure 140. Sabre cut or superior approach used for repair of ruptures of the rotator cuff. Skin incision outlined as well as the acromion.

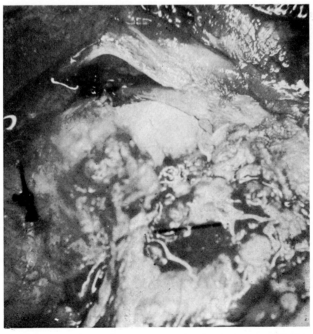

Figure 141. Exposure of shoulder reveals large irregular tear of the cuff.

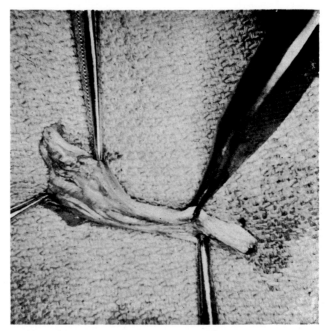

Figure 142. Intra-articular portion of long head of the biceps is partially sectioned longitudinally in a book-like fashion. (Courtesy *Arch Surgery, 102*:483–485, May 1971, Copyright 1971, AMA).

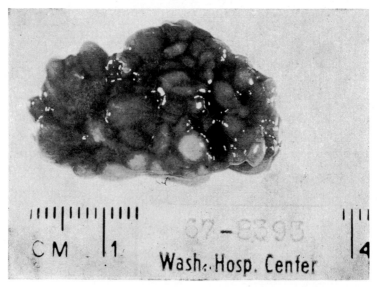

Figure 143. Gross appearance of the specimen taken from the subdeltoid bursa with a pigmented villonodular synovitis.

groove. The distal portion of the biceps is fixed in the bicipital groove in the usual manner. The intraarticular portion of the biceps is then sectioned in a book-like fashion (Fig. 142). This provides a graft wide enough to cover the humeral head and close the shoulder joint. The free graft, with the glistening surface facing the joint, is sutured to the cuff edges with interrupted braided silk or polyester fiber suture as seen in Figure 139. Any excess graft is discarded. After the last suture has been placed we should have a watertight capsule. This can be tested by injecting sterile saline into the joint away from the suture lines. If there is no leakage then we can proceed with the final closure, otherwise, one or two additional sutures may be placed wherever any leakage is observed. The bursa is resutured unless it is unusually thickened or diseased. If so, it is discarded. I prefer to leave the bursa as I believe it helps to maintain the gliding mechanism between the cuff and deltoid. After replacing the deltoid on the acromion, the skin is closed and a stockinette or an Unna's type Velpeau dressing is applied. On the first postoperative day the patient is

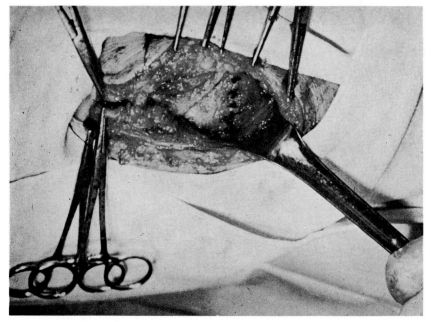

Figure 144. End-to-end suture of rupture of the rotator cuff. (Courtesy *Arch Surgery, 102:*483–485, May 1971, Copyright 1971, AMA).

encouraged to shrug or elevate his shoulders about ten times every two hours. This helps prevent the formation of any adhesions between the deltoid, bursa and cuff. This is a helpful exercise since the deltoid tends to contract somewhat when one shrugs or elevates their shoulders. After three weeks the stockinette Velpeau dressing is removed and the arm placed in a sling for one week. The patient is started on pendulum exercises. After discarding the sling, full range of motion of the shoulder is encouraged.

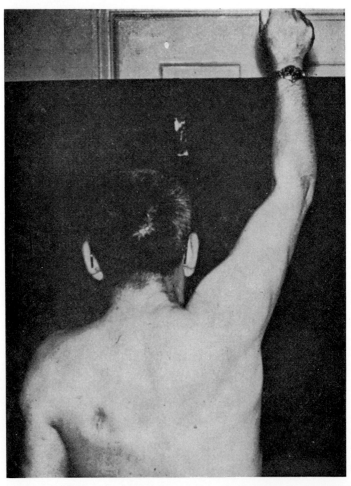

Figure 145. Abduction of 150 degrees after routine repair of tear of the rotator cuff.

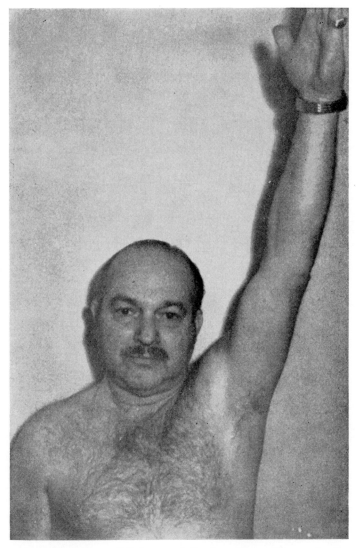

Figure 146. Abduction to 170 degrees following side-to-side repair of rotator cuff seven months post-operatively.

Two patients had a chronic villonodular synovitis or bursitis of the subdeltoid bursa (Fig. 143) which were confirmed by microscopic examination. It is possible that the lesion may have been the underlying cause of the cuff rupture through pressure erosion as neither patient gave any history of injury. Following removal

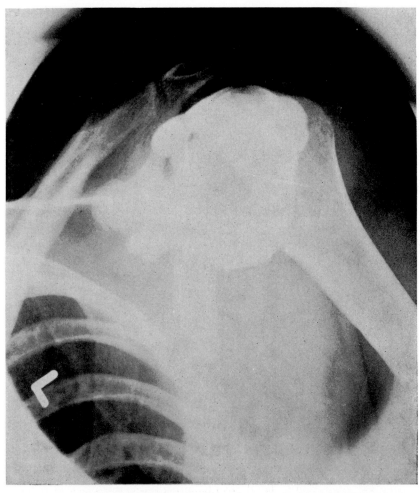

Figure 147. Arthrogram of shoulder following side-to-side repair of rupture of rotator cuff six months post-operatively. Appearance of arthrogram is normal.

of the lesional tissue, the rupture in each case was repaired by approximating the edges side to side with braided silk sutures.

In one case the long head of the biceps had become displaced medially out of the bicipital groove and eroded the cuff from within. Repair of the tear in this instance was relatively simple once the intraarticular portion of the biceps was resected, discarded and the distal portion of the biceps fixed in the bicipital groove.

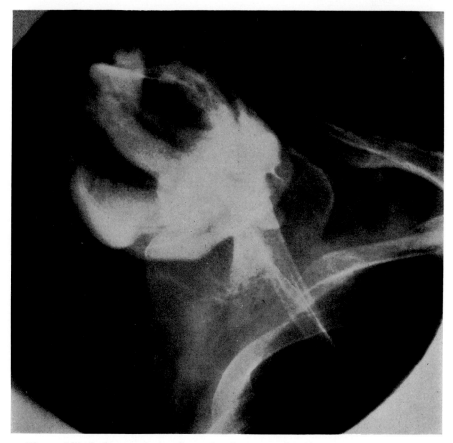

Figure 148. Arthrography performed prior to surgery. Arthrogram taken with the arm in some abduction. Note dye in the subdeltoid bursa.

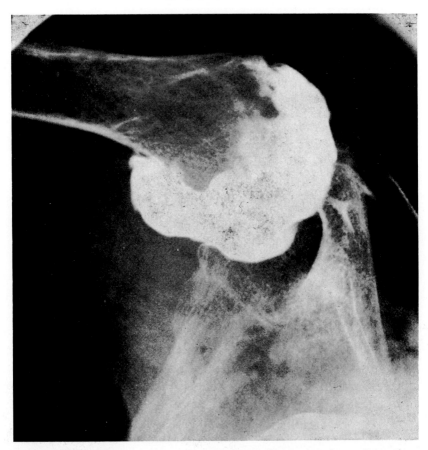

Figure 149. Arthrogram taken two and one half months after using a free biceps graft to repair a rupture of the rotator cuff. The arm is in the same abducted position as in Figure 148. No dye is visualized in the subdeltoid bursa.

End Results of Operative Repair of Chronic Ruptures of the Rotator Cuff

The functional results of the cuff repairs sutured end to end or side to side were satisfactory (Fig. 144). The constant pain was relieved and the majority of the patients had only a slight discomfort in the shoulder. Active abduction varied from 150 degrees to 175 degrees (Figs. 145, 146). An arthrogram performed on a

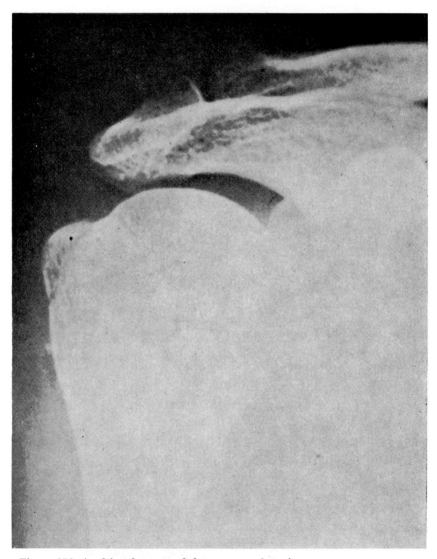

Figure 150. Avulsion fracture of the greater tuberosity.

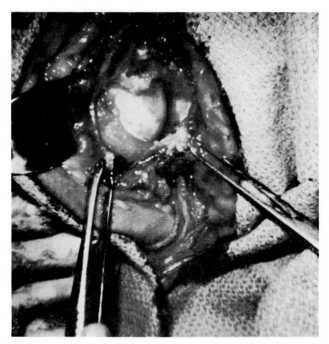

Figure 151. Rupture of the rotator cuff. The tuberosity is bare as a result of the avulsion of the tendons of the external rotators from their sites of insertion.

shoulder following a side to side repair of a rupture six months previously revealed a normal arthrogram (Fig. 147).

The end results of the cases where a free biceps tendon graft was used were quite good. Active abduction ranged from 150 degrees to 175 degrees. Pain was greatly relieved in these patients and each was able to sleep without resorting to any regular medication. One patient was kind enough to allow me to perform an arthrogram two and one-half months after surgery (Figs. 148, 149). The film was taken with the arm in the same abducted position as before surgery and, it revealed no extravasation of dye in the subdeltoid bursa. This was good evidence that the free biceps graft had closed the gap in the cuff and was containing the solution within the joint cavity.

Recently we have had some cases where the cuff edges were so retracted we could not cover the humeral head even with the use

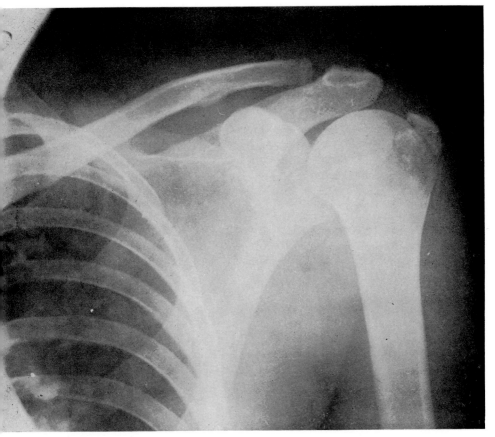

Figure 152. An avulsion fracture of the greater tuberosity with only a slight displacement of the fragment.

of a free biceps tendon graft. In these instances we have used large pieces of freeze-dried rotator cuff grafts to close the defect over the humeral head. The results to date have been encouraging.

AVULSION FRACTURES OF THE GREATER TUBEROSITY

Fractures of the greater tuberosity may, at times, appear to be a somewhat innocuous lesion, but patients may have an associated rupture with this injury. Since the external rotator tendons insert on this bony prominence they are vulnerable to a tear if the tuberosity is fractured. This is particularly true in patients past the middle age.

Figure 150 is a roentgenogram of a fifty-one-year-old male who injured his right shoulder about three months previously. His arm was kept in a sling for three weeks. He was then encouraged to use his arm. The pain in his shoulder persisted and, when he was seen, his abduction was 145 degrees. An arthrogram revealed dye in the subdeltoid bursa. At operation a rupture was easily seen (Fig. 151). The greater tuberosity was bare where the external rotators had pulled off. Figure 152 reveals another avulsion fracture of the greater tuberosity. This patient also had clinical signs of a rupture, namely pain and some limitation of abduction. Arthrography confirmed the diagnosis and at operation the bare tuberosity was easily seen (Fig. 153). The rupture was repaired, fixing the external rotator tendons into the tuberosity by passing the sutures through drill holes made below the tuberosity.

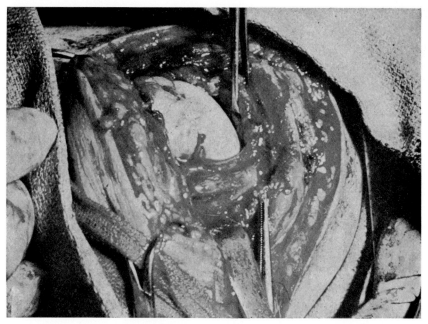

Figure 153. Greater tuberosity is completely bare as the tendons have been completely avulsed and retracted.

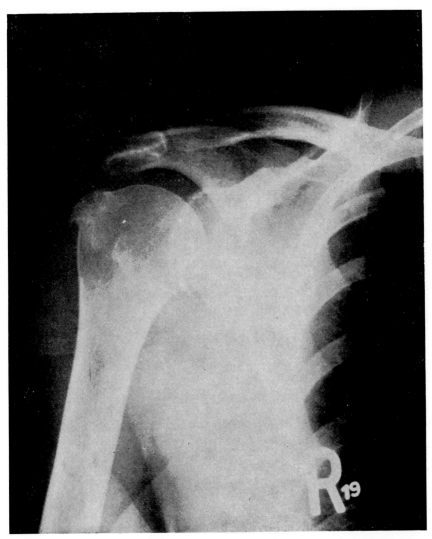

Figure 154. Fracture of the Greater Tuberosity seen seven months after injury. Because of the innocuous appearance of the fracture little attention was paid to her complaints of persistent pain.

Figure 154 is the roentgenographic appearance of the right shoulder of a sixty-one-year-old female who fell and injured her shoulder seven months prior to the time I saw her. Her arm was kept in a sling for three weeks. Afterwards she was encouraged to use her arm. Although her motion was satisfactory, abduction being 150 degrees, her main complaint was persistent pain. An arthrogram revealed dye in the subdeltoid bursa (Fig. 155). On the axillary view one can see the dye in the bursa outlined in a half-moon manner (Fig. 156). At operation, the humeral head was exposed and one could also see the bare appearance of the greater tuberosity (Fig. 157).

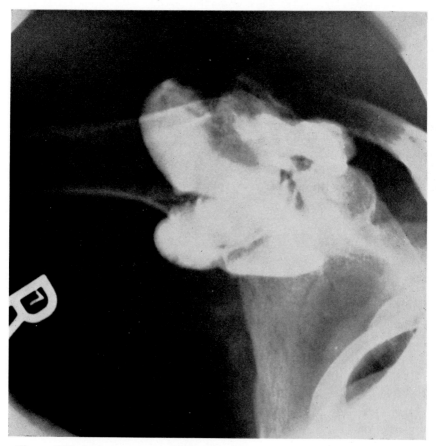

Figure 155. Arthrogram reveals dye in the subdeltoid bursa with the arm in some abduction.

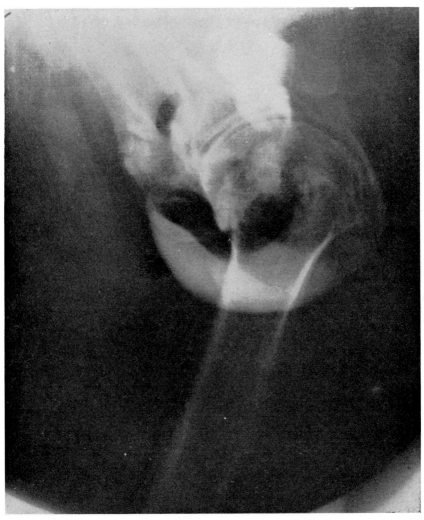

Figure 156. Axillary view of the arthrogram shows the dye in the subdeltoid bursa outlined in a half-moon manner.

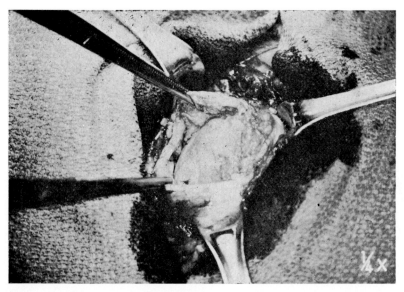

Figure 157. Humeral head exposed by retracting the cuff edges. The greater tuberosity is stripped of its attachments.

It is quite evident that avulsion fractures should be kept under observation for some time past the healing period of the fracture. If pain persists, arthrography is indicated to rule out a rupture even though the patient may have fairly good abduction motion in the shoulder.

Chapter Five

LESIONS OF THE
BICEPS TENDON

LESIONS OF THE BICEPS TENDONS were considered a rather uncommon condition. Ruptures of the long head of the biceps seemed to be the only lesion that warranted consideration and treatment. Arthrography has convinced me of two other pathological conditions that can result in a definite shoulder disability. The more frequent one is a tenosynovitis of the sheath of the long head of the biceps and the less common one is the medial displacement or subluxation of the biceps tendon out of the bicipital groove.

The following cases illustrate these problems:

A fifty-five-year-old female complained of left shoulder pain of six months' duration. There was no definite history of an injury although her work required opening and closing file cabinets frequently. Shoulder motion was quite good but tenderness was elicited over the bicipital groove. The biceps resistance test was positive. An arthrogram revealed dilatation and irregularity of the biceps sheath (Fig. 158). On the bicipital groove view the sheath was dilated and distended greater than normal (Fig. 159). At operation the biceps sheath was found to be thickened and irregular. The intraarticular portion of the tendon was resected and the distal portion was fixed in the bicipital groove.

A sixty-four-year-old female was seen because of pain in her right shoulder for a period of about eight months. She worked as a telephone operator on a switch board. The clinical findings were suggestive of a biceps tenosynovitis. Arthrography was performed after conservative treatment had failed. It revealed a thinning proximally of the biceps sheath while distally the sheath was distended and irregular (Fig. 160). At operation the pathologic findings confirmed those of the arthrograms. Actually the proximal portion of the sheath was thicker than visualized on the arthrograms.

157

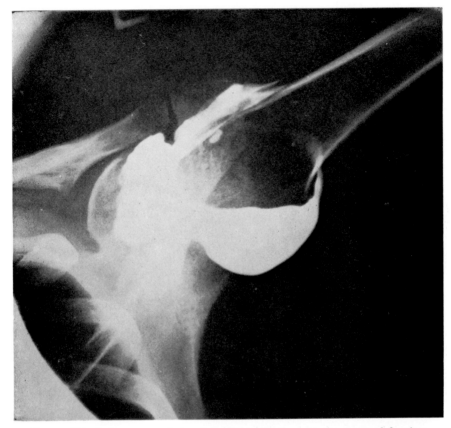

Figure 158. Arthrogram of the shoulder with the arm in some abduction. Tendon sheath is dilated and irregular suggestive of a tenosynovitis of the biceps sheath.

A male, sixty-six years of age, fell on his outstretched left arm three months prior to the time of my examination. He had persistent pain but his shoulder motions were within normal limits. Arthrograms revealed marked dilatation and irregularity of the biceps sheath distally (Fig. 161). A notch was seen just medial to the greater tuberosity where this area impinged against the acromion when he fell on his outstretched arm. When the arm was abducted dye was seen escaping into the subdeltoid bursa and the biceps sheath was distended along its entire length (Fig. 162). Exposure of the joint revealed the biceps sheath thickened and dilated with a small tear found in the supraspinatus tendon just proximal to its insertion. The tear was easily repaired after the biceps tendon was resected proximally and the distal

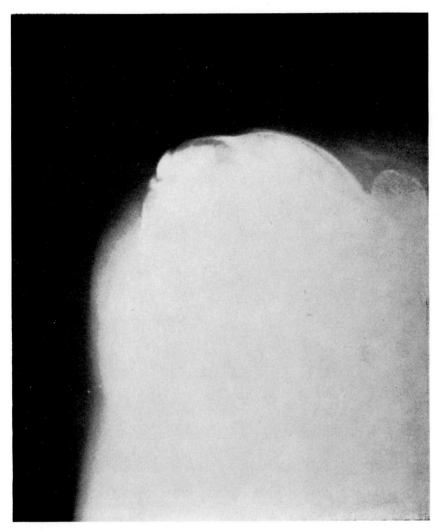

Figure 159. Bicipital groove view of an arthrogram. Biceps sheath is greatly dilated and distended.

portion fixed in the bicipital groove. The functional result after surgery was excellent.

A fifty-seven-year-old female was pulling a drawer open and felt a sudden tearing feeling in her left shoulder. The clinical examination revealed an obvious rupture of the biceps tendon proximally. The arthrogram showed dye extravasating distally out of the sheath where

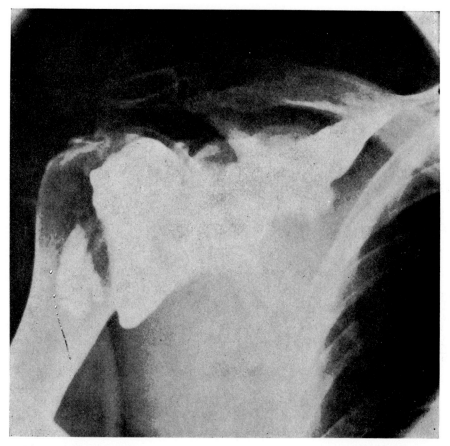

Figure 160. Observe the thinning of the proximal portion of the biceps sheath and the distension and irregularity of the sheath distally.

the tendon had pulled through it (Figs. 163, 164). Although this is a frequent picture seen in ruptures of the long head of the biceps, I have also seen arthrograms where the biceps sheath is not outlined at all in biceps ruptures. This is the result of hemorrhage in the sheath with clot formation which prevents extravasation of the dye into the sheath.

A twenty-three-year-old male developed pain in his right shoulder after playing basketball about six weeks prior to my examination. The shoulder motions were good but there was tenderness over the bicipital groove. The patient had pain over the groove when the arm was held in forward flexion against resistance. The arthrogram revealed dilatation and prolongation of the biceps sheath (Fig. 165). In addition,

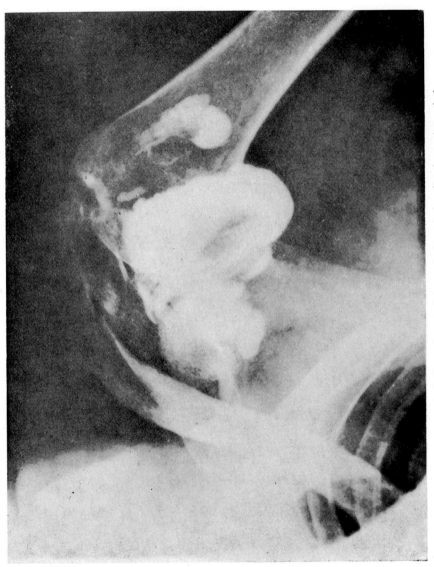

Figure 161. Marked distension and irregularity of the distal portion of the biceps sheath is seen. The notch in the humeral head just medial to the greater tuberosity suggested the possibility of a cuff tear.

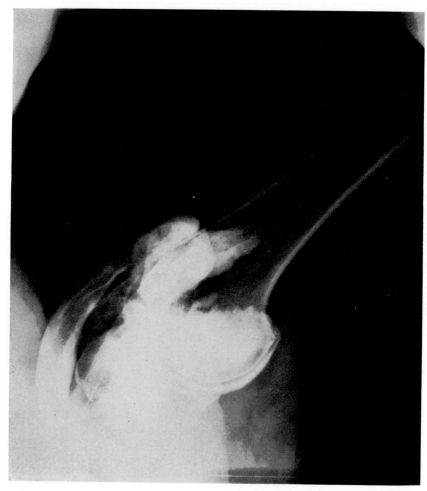

Figure 162. Arthrogram with the arm in some abduction. Dye seen in the subdeltoid bursa and the biceps sheath is fully distended along its entire length. A tear in the supraspinatus tendon as well as the distended and thickened sheath were found at operation.

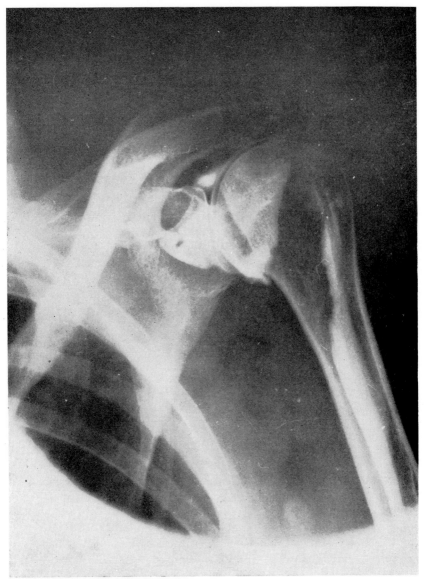

Figure 163. Arthrogram of a rupture of the Biceps Tendon. There is extravasation of dye out of the biceps sheath extending down the distal part of the humerus.

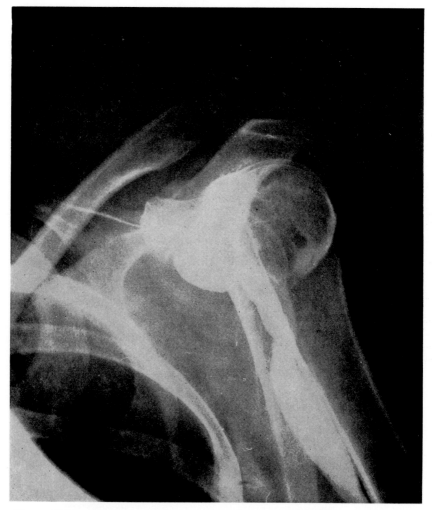

Figure 164. Arthrogram of the same case seen in Figure 163 with the arm held in internal rotation.

there was very little visualization of the dye at the origin of the tendon near the supraglenoid tuberosity. Under treatment consisting of avoiding heavy lifting and restricted activity, particularly refraining from playing basketball, this patient recovered in three weeks' time.

A sixty-one-year-old electrician was pulling and jerking some heavy wire when he felt a snapping sensation and pain in his shoulder. This feeling, with the accompanying pain, would recur whenever he did

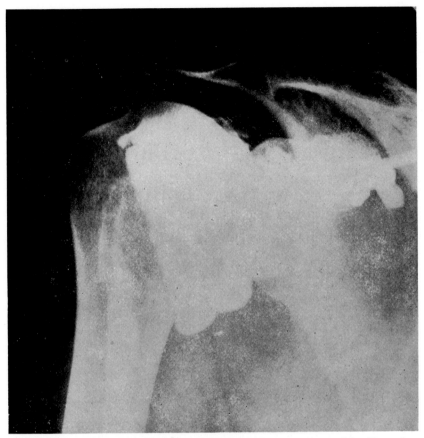

Figure 165. Arthrogram of a patient with a biceps tenosynovitis. Note the dilatation and prolongation of the biceps sheath. The sheath is not outlined well near the origin of the tendon at the supraglenoid tuberosity.

any pulling or lifting. When seen about a month after his injury he described his feelings as "my shoulder seems to jump out of place." There was tenderness over the bicipital groove. The biceps tendon could be rolled under the examiner's finger at the groove. Forward flexion against resistance gave the patient pain over the bicipital groove area. An arthrogram in the anterior-posterior view revealed no real visualization of the biceps sheath. There was an elevation of the capsule and sheath just distal to the supraglenoid tuberosity (Fig. 166). On the bicipital groove view one notes the displacement medially of the biceps within its sheath (Fig. 167). At operation the biceps tendon was displaced medially out of the groove.

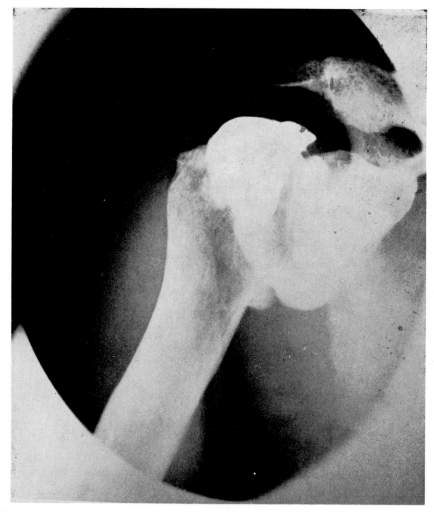

Figure 166. Arthrogram reveals almost complete absence of the biceps sheath although there is some elevation of the capsule and sheath noted superiorly and lateral to the supraglenoid tuberosity.

Another illustration of a displaced biceps tendon was seen in a fifty-year-old-male whose right arm was pulled backward quite severely in an altercation. He developed pain immediately over the upper anterior region of the arm. When seen six weeks after injury he had pain over the bicipital groove area upon full forward flexion against resistance as well as in backward extension. An arthrogram revealed dilatation

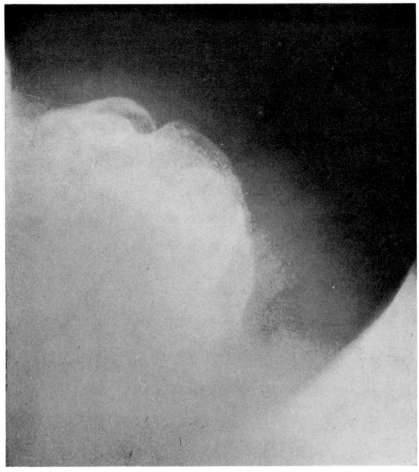

Figure 167. The bicipital groove view shows displacement medially of the biceps tendon within its sheath.

of the distal portion of the biceps sheath with a broadening of the sheath as it passed into the shoulder capsule (Fig. 168). When the arm was abducted the sheath appeared to be elevated from the upper humeral shaft, suggestive of a displaced biceps tendon (Fig. 169). The axillary view does not show the normal prolongation of the sheath through the bicipital groove but it appears displaced below the lesser tuberosity (Fig. 170). At operation the tendon was found to be displaced medially out of the intertubercular groove.

A young man, seventeen years of age, was seen complaining that he "feels like his left shoulder dislocates." He stated that in the football

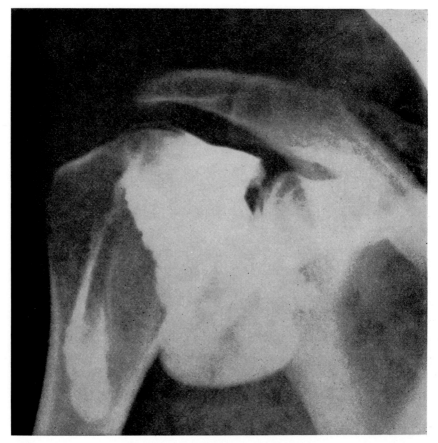

Figure 168. Arthrogram of right shoulder reveals a dilated biceps sheath distally and a widening of the nipple-like sheath as the tendon enters the joint capsule.

season the previous year his shoulder would hurt whenever he played. He recalled no specific injury. After the season was over his shoulder continued to bother him only when it was jarred. The following fall he started to play football again and his shoulder began to give him more pain. He also thought that the shoulder would dislocate, but he was not sure because of the pads on his shoulders. At times he could not move his arm except with the use of his other hand and then the shoulder would seem to snap into place. This happened quite often during the football season and occasionally while he was sleeping. Upon clinical examination the motions of the left shoulder were good. Tenderness was elicited over the bicipital groove. In addition, he had

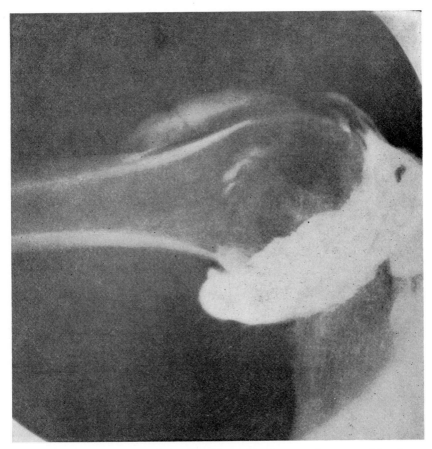

Figure 169. Arthrogram of the shoulder with the arm in some abduction. The biceps sheath does not lie close to the groove as it should normally but is somewhat elevated above the cortical border.

pain over the bicipital groove when the arm was flexed forward against resistance. He could not supinate the pronated forearm against resistance without pain. An arthrogram revealed irregularity and some elevation of the biceps sheath (Fig. 171). It was felt that the patient had a dislocating biceps tendon. At operation the tendon was displaced medially. It also was rather soft and the sheath was red and mushy. The intraarticular portion of the tendon was resected and the distal portion was fixed in the bicipital groove. Following the operation the feeling of the shoulder going out of the joint had disappeared. The functional result was quite good.

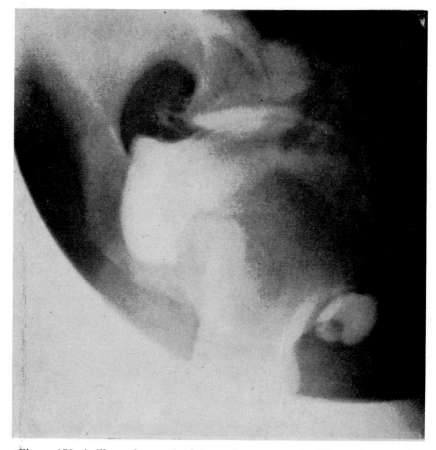

Figure 170. Axillary view again fails to demonstrate the biceps sheath lying within the confines of the groove but remains well outlined below the lesser tuberosity.

A twenty-seven-year-old male was seen complaining of his right shoulder "going out of place." He recalled no definite injury except that he had this feeling whenever he played basketball. This would occur if he would throw with his arm in the abducted position. The shoulder would seem to slip back in place when he put the arm down and "juggled and rotated it." The motions of the shoulder were good but there was definite tenderness over the bicipital groove and pain in forward flexion of the arm against resistance. An arthrogram revealed a medial displacement of the biceps tendon which is seen on the bicipital groove view (Fig. 172). Exposure of the shoulder at operation confirmed the diagnosis of the displacement of the biceps

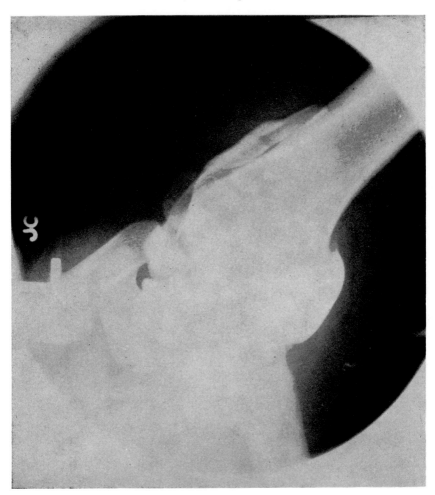

Figure 171. Arthrogram taken with the arm in some abduction reveals an irregular outline of the biceps sheath. It also appears to be somewhat elevated. A dislocating biceps tendon was suspected.

tendon. The distal portion of the tendon was fixed in the bicipital groove after the intraarticular portion had been resected. The patient did well and had no further difficulty while playing basketball.

A fifty-year-old male who had been playing handball almost daily since his youth developed a sudden pain in his left shoulder when he fell on the shoulder while wrestling. He continued this sport despite his discomfort until suddenly he had so much pain he could not continue with the game. He tried home remedies for about six weeks.

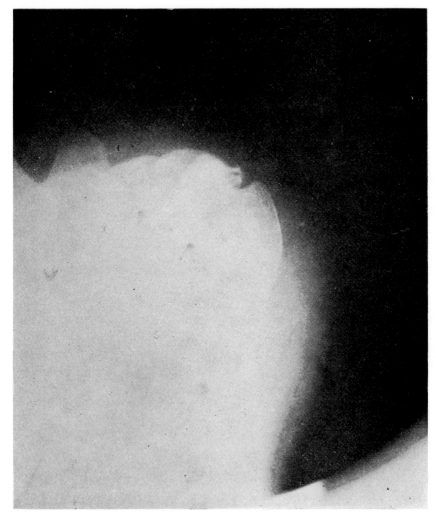

Figure 172. Bicipital groove view of an arthrogram of the right shoulder. There is a definite medial displacement of the biceps sheath. A displaced long head of the biceps was found at operation.

At the time of my examination active abduction was 110 degrees. He had pain when the arm was abducted with the palm down. There was tenderness over the bicipital groove as well as behind the greater tuberosity. The patient had weakness in abduction as well as forward flexion against resistance. An arthrogram revealed dye in the subdeltoid bursa as well as a definite displacement of the biceps sheath

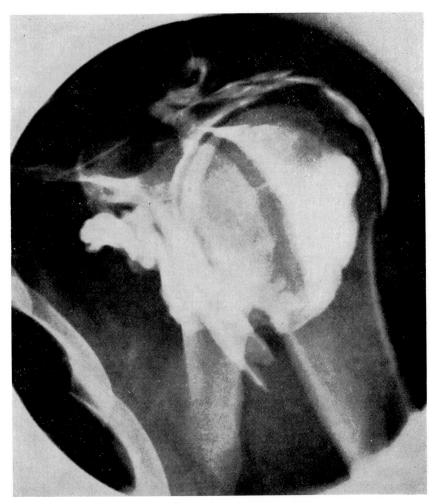

Figure 173. Arthrogram reveals dye in the subdeltoid bursa indicative of a rupture but also a definite medial displacement of the biceps sheath.

medially (Figs. 173, 174). At operation there was a massive rupture of the entire rotator cuff with the subscapularis tendon completely torn from its attachment to the lesser tuberosity. Both tuberosities were bare and the cuff edges were markedly retracted and irregular. In addition, the biceps tendon was displaced medially, lying over the rim of the glenoid. The tendon was so soft and attenuated it could not be used as a free graft for the repair. Closure of the capsule was obtained only after tedious and prolonged dissection to free the cuff

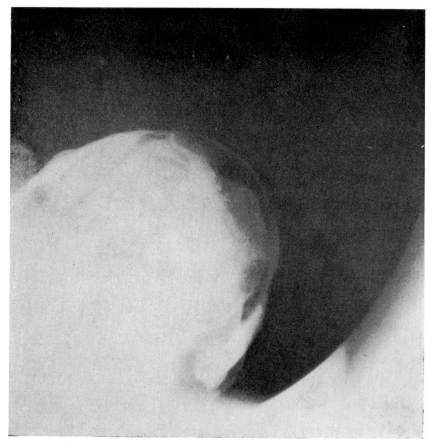

Figure 174. Bicipital groove view of the arthrogram on the shoulder seen in Figure 173 shows a circular outline of dye about the humeral head as well as a medial displacement of the biceps sheath.

from the adherent surrounding structures. Although the patient was relieved of much of his pain, active abduction was only 85 degrees after two months. This case again proved the necessity of making a diagnosis of a rupture early and confirming the diagnosis by an arthrogram. If surgical repair is performed early the chances for a good result are enhanced.

A chef, fifty-eight years of age, fell over an object on the floor injuring his right shoulder. He went to a workmen's compensation clinic where he was X-rayed. They revealed no evidence of a fracture or dislocation about the shoulder. He was given physical therapy to the shoulder without relief. He was referred to an orthopedic surgeon

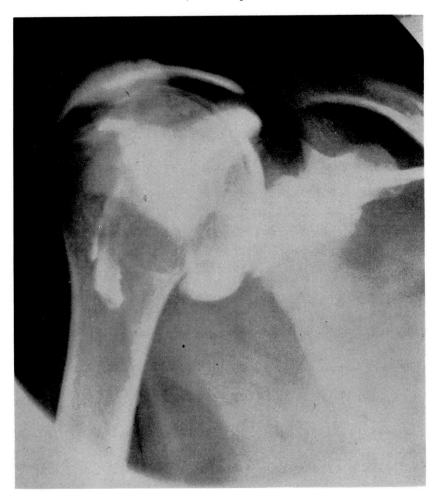

Figure 175. Arthrogram reveals dye in the subdeltoid bursa pathognomonic of a rupture. A poor outline of the biceps sheath proximally with distension and irregularity of the sheath distally is indicative of biceps pathology.

after a month who continued with conservative treatment. No arthrograms were suggested or ordered. When seen by me eight months later the patient still had pain and could only abduct his arm to 90 degrees in the forward plane. An arthrogram was done. It revealed dye in the subdeltoid bursa (Figs. 175, 176). Even the routine films suggested the possibility of two lesions (Figs. 177, 178). At operation performed three weeks later, the cuff had three small tears in addition to a larger one overlying the biceps tendon. Further exposure of the biceps tendon

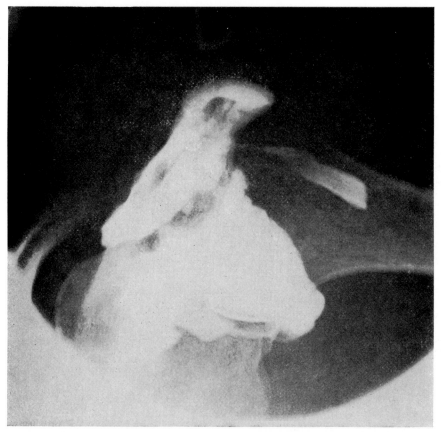

Figure 176. Arthrogram with the arm in some abduction. The dye has fully distended the subdeltoid bursa and the proximal portion of the biceps sheath is not visualized well.

revealed the sheath to be inflammed, thickened and nodular, similar to a chronic villonodular synovitis. The tendon was excised, the sheath removed and the distal portion fixed in the bicipital groove. The tears in the cuff were repaired without difficulty. The end result in this case was good. The patient returned to work, pain was minimal and the motions of the shoulder were excellent.

It has been suggested that in the repair of an acute rupture of the long head of the biceps tendon or subluxation of the biceps tendon out of the bicipital groove, the tendon should be transferred to the coracoid process and plicated to the short head. The reason given for doing this type of procedure was that consider-

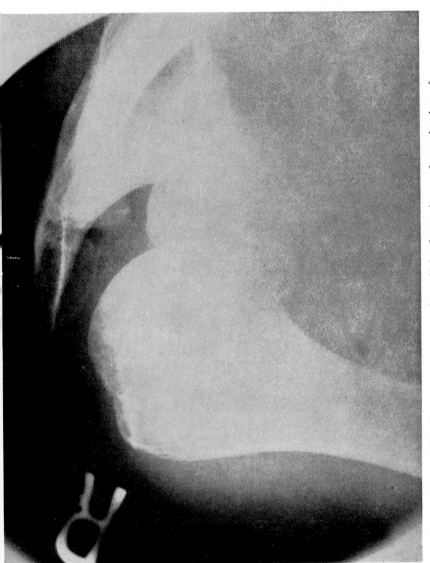

Figure 177. Roentgenogram reveals a slight depression and roughening of the head with some cystic changes just medial to the greater tuberosity which could have resulted from an impingement of the head against the acromion when the patient fell on his outstretched arm.

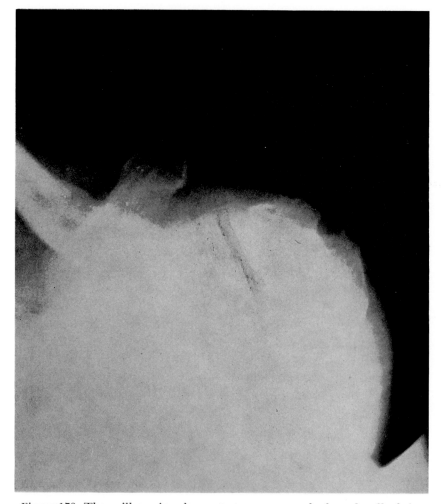

Figure 178. The axillary view demonstrates a spur at the lateral wall of the bicipital groove. This bony spur could have been the cause of the biceps tenosynovitis which was found at operation.

able power of flexion at the shoulder would be lost and there would be a decrease in flexion and supination of the forearm. This has not been my experience. Resecting the proximal portion of the biceps with fixation of the distal portion into the bicipital groove has not altered the strength of flexion of the shoulder or elbow nor weakened supination of the forearm.

DISLOCATIONS OF THE SHOULDER

ARTHROGRAPHY can be a valuable adjunct in the diagnosis and management of various types of dislocations of the shoulder. In a recurrent dislocation it can outline the anterior pouch, which is the result of the separation of the capsule or a stripping of the periosteum from the anterior surface of the neck of the scapula with or without a detachment of the glenoid labrum. The redundancy or increased laxity of the posterior capsule can also be visualized by arthrography in cases of recurrent posterior subluxation of the humeral head. Arthrograms can also demonstrate the bow-stringing of the capsule across the glenoid in old unreduced anterior or posterior dislocations.

Dislocations of the shoulder or dislocations with fracture of the greater tuberosity which may result in a rupture of the musculotendinous cuff has been discussed in Chapter 4 entitled "Ruptures of the Rotator Cuff."

RECURRENT ANTERIOR DISLOCATIONS

Although the bony defect in the posterolateral surface of the head of the humerus, the compression fracture or the Hill-Sachs lesion, can be demonstrated by radiological examination using special projection techniques, arthrograms will reveal the soft tissue lesions, namely the increased joint capacity, the anterior capsular pouch or stripping of the capsule from the neck of the scapula anteriorly. The surgeon frequently will see a patient with a history of a recurrent dislocation but he will seldom see him with the shoulder dislocated. Arthrography may be of help in determining the type of lesion present and, in turn, may influ-

ence the surgeon in his selection of the proper operative procedure for correction of the basic problems noted.

A twenty-three-year-old medical student gave a history of recurrent
dislocations of his right shoulder following an original dislocation
playing basketball two years previously. Arthrograms taken of both
shoulders in the same position revealed some laxity of the dependent

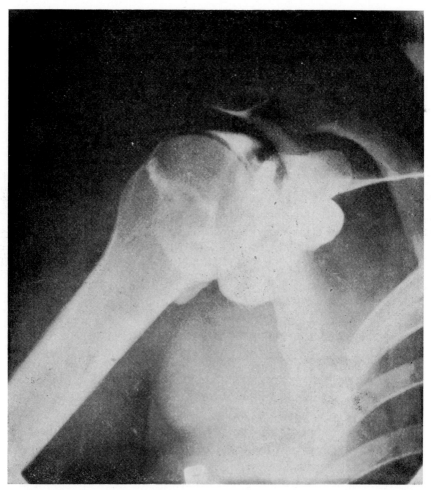

Figure 179. Arthrogram of the right shoulder of a patient with a history of
a recurrent dislocation. Note the laxity of the dependent fold and the
presence of dye over the anterior surface of the neck of the scapula.

fold as compared to the left shoulder (Figs. 179, 180). Dye was seen over the anterior surface of the neck of the scapula as the result of the capsular stripping from the neck. Repair by the Putti-Platt procedure would be the operation of choice. This was done and the end result was excellent.

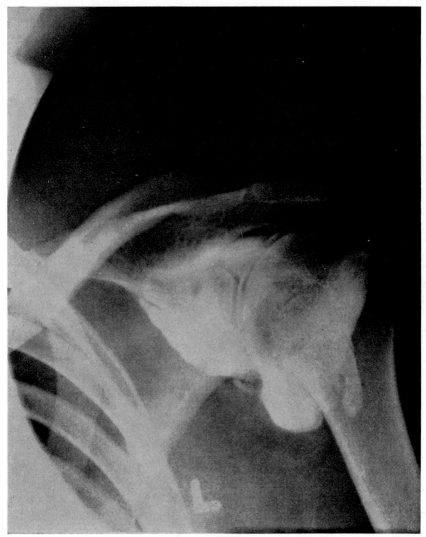

Figure 180. Normal arthrogram of the left shoulder. No redundancy of the inferior capsule is seen and very little dye is present over the anterior-inferior surface of the scapular neck.

A young man, twenty-two years of age, was seen following frequent episodes of recurrent dislocations of the left shoulder after a football injury sustained thirty months previously. Arthrograms of the left shoulder revealed an enlarged capsule inferiorly with dye present over the neck of the scapula to a greater degree than in the right shoulder (Figs. 181, 182). Axillary views of the arthrograms show stripping of the periosteum and capsule from the scapular neck anteriorly close to the glenoid labrum (Fig. 183). Compare this with the normal arthrogram of the right shoulder (Fig. 184). A Bankart procedure was performed on this patient as an anterior detachment of the glenoid

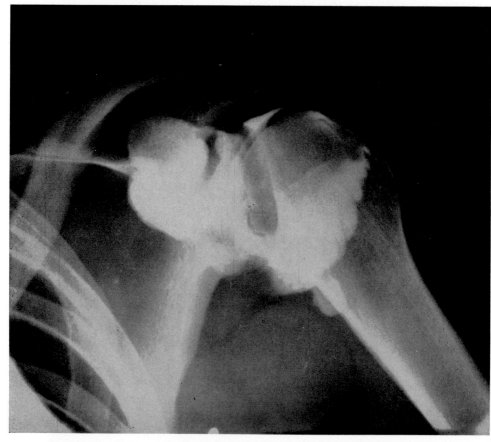

Figure 181. Arthrogram of the left shoulder reveals a relaxed capsule inferiorly. Note dye present over the scapular neck anteriorly to a greater degree than in the right shoulder (Fig. 182).

labrum was found in addition to the anterior pouch. Suturing of the capsule to the bony rim of the glenoid corrected the pathology.

The laxity and redundancy of the capsule in recurrent dislocations of the shoulder is illustrated well in the following case:

A thirty-six-year-old male was seen with a dislocation of his right shoulder. Originally he had dislocated his shoulder about three years previously. Since that time he had had many episodes of dislocation. Arthrography was done with the shoulder out of joint (Figs. 185, 186).

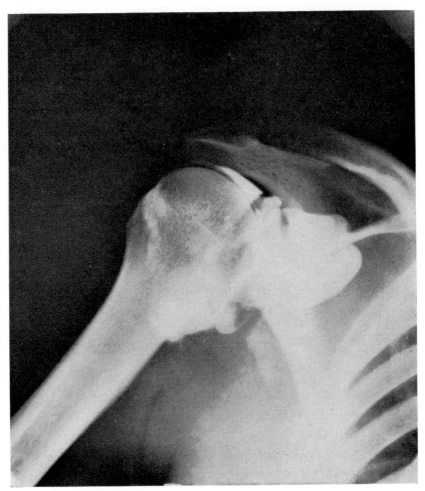

Figure 182. Arthrogram of a normal shoulder on the right side.

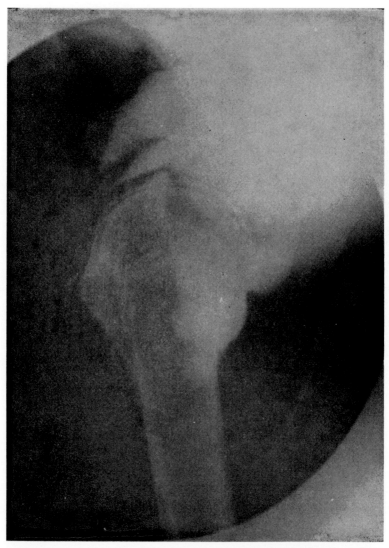

Figure 183. Axillary view of arthrogram of the left shoulder. There is stripping of the periosteum and capsule from the neck of the scapula anteriorly close to the glenoid rim suggesting the existence of a Bankart lesion. Compare with Figure 184.

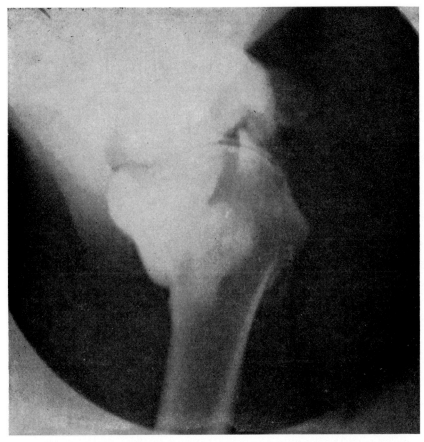

Figure 184. Axillary view of arthrogram of the right shoulder which is normal.

On the A-P view there was definite laxity of the capsule (Fig. 187). The dislocation was an intraarticular lesion as the rotator cuff was intact without any extravasation of dye. On the axillary view (Fig. 188) the capsule could be seen bow-stringing across the glenoid. In old unreduced dislocations of the shoulder the bow-stringing of the capsule across the glenoid is the main obstacle in the reduction of chronic dislocations.

RECURRENT POSTERIOR SUBLUXATIONS
OR DISLOCATIONS

The clinical findings are not as definite as in a true posterior dislocation since the posterior displacement of the humeral head

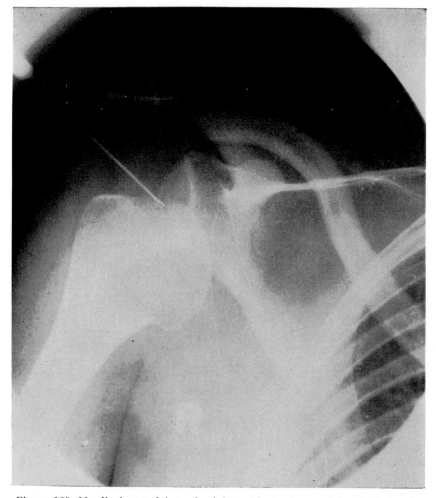

Figure 185. Needle inserted into the joint with the humeral head displaced anteriorly and inferiorly.

is seldom complete. One may elicit a history of the shoulder "going out of joint" when the arm is flexed forward, internally rotated and adducted. The head of the humerus will slip off the posterior rim of the glenoid becoming displaced as a result of a relaxed posterior capsule. When it engages the posterior glenoid rim, the patient may be able to reduce the subluxation himself.

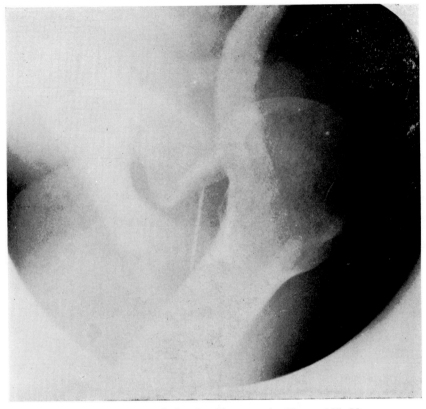

Figure 186. Axillary view of the shoulder seen in Figure 185. Note proper placement of the needle.

as there may be only a rather shallow groove or defect in the humeral head.

Axillary views of the shoulder clearly demonstrate how the head slips posteriorly (Figs. 189, 190). Arthrograms show a relaxed posterior capsule in the normal position (Fig. 191) but when the head slips backwards the capsule is distended further posteriorly while the dye is pushed anteriorly (Fig. 192).

Another patient with a recurrent posterior subluxation presented a normal appearance on the axillary view (Fig. 193) but a definite posterior displacement of the head when the patient forward flexed his arm and pushed against resistance (Fig. 194). Arthrograms revealed

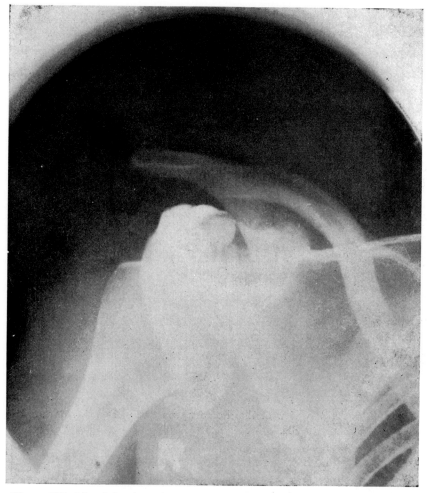

Figure 187. After injection of 16 cc of dye. Observe the marked laxity of the shoulder capsule. Capsule is intact as no dye is seen extravasating from the joint.

a noticeably relaxed posterior capsule in the normal position (Fig. 195). The head filled the posterior capsular space when subluxated posteriorly and the dye occupied the empty space opposite the glenoid (Fig. 196).

The arthrograms of the right shoulder of a twenty-six-year-old male with a history of a recurrent subluxation of about two year's duration

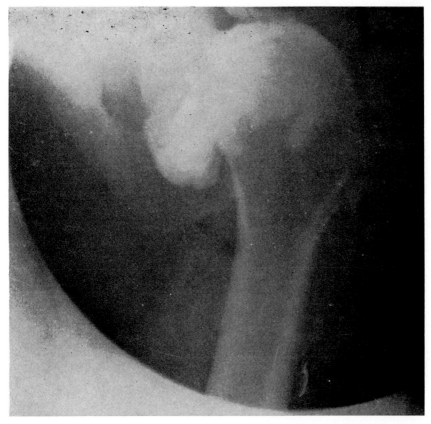

Figure 188. Axillary view of the arthrogram. Capsule is seen bow-stringing across the glenoid. No extra-articular escaping of dye is visualized.

revealed a large subscapularis bursa anteriorly (Fig. 197) when the head was in the joint. When the head was displaced posteriorly, it occupied the distended capsule posteriorly, while the capsule was bow-stringing across the glenoid. The dye from the subscapularis bursa was now seen in the space opposite the glenoid (Fig. 198).

An arthrogram of a left shoulder taken with the head subluxated posteriorly would seem to indicate that the biceps tendon had become displaced medially (Fig. 199). This false impression was created by the marked internal rotation of the humerus. The axillary view showed the biceps in normal rela-

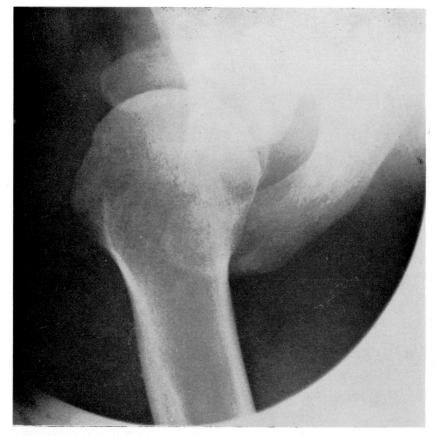

Figure 189. A case of recurrent posterior subluxation of the shoulder. Axillary view taken with the humeral head in a normal position.

tionship with the humerus (Fig. 200). The bow-stringing of the capsule across the glenoid is readily seen.

The majority of recurrent posterior subluxations can be repaired by a Putti-Platt type of operation through a posterior approach imbricating the capsule after roughening the posterior portion of the scapular neck.

OLD UNREDUCED DISLOCATIONS OF THE SHOULDER

The management of old unreduced dislocations of the shoulder, whether the treatment was of the conservative or the opera-

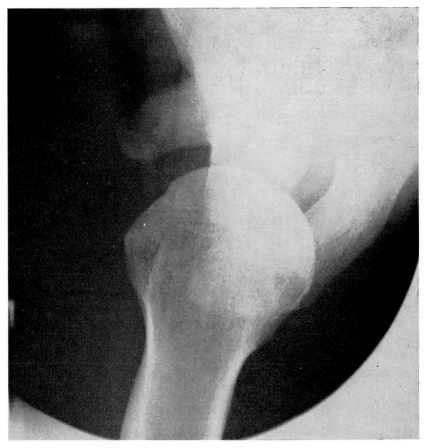

Figure 190. Axillary view taken when the head has been displaced posteriorly.

tive type, has been frequently unsatisfactory. Our investigations have shown that there are many obstacles encountered at operation. There was difficulty in replacing the humeral head because of fibrosis and shortening of the muscles as well as contracture and bow-stringing of the capsule across the glenoid cavity. Frequently there was notching or wedging of the head of the humerus at the point of impingement on the glenoid, at times, the presence of scar tissue in the glenoid fossa, and finally, the difficulty in maintaining the reduction after the shoulder had been reduced. The main obstacle was the bow-stringing of the capsule across the glenoid, the others were the end result of this process.

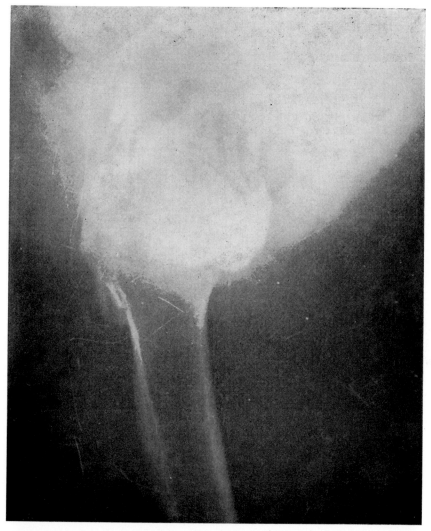

Figure 191. On the arthrogram a redundant posterior capsule is seen with the head in the normal position.

The pathological process of this bow-stringing can be explained best by the three sketches shown. The first sketch shows the normal relationship of the capsule (Fig. 201). Notice the firm attachment of the capsule to the anterior surface of the neck of the scapula while there is some redundancy of the capsule

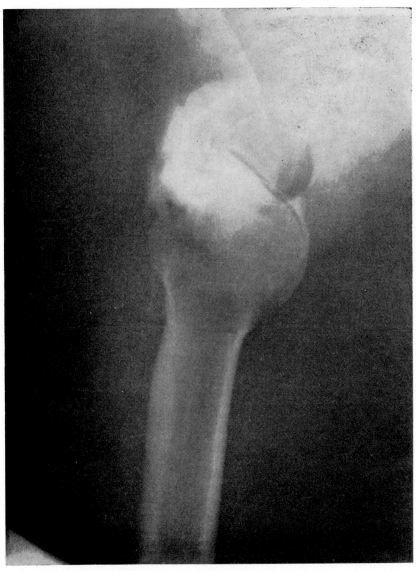

Figure 192. When the head subluxates posteriorly notice how the capsule is displaced backward and the dye pushed anteriorly.

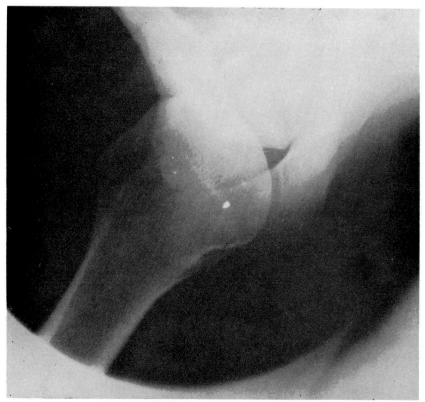

Figure 193. Axillary view reveals head in a normal position.

posteriorly. The relationship of the capsule is changed greatly when the head is dislocated anteriorly and remains unreduced for a period of three weeks or more. With the capsule remaining bow-stringing across the glenoid, the posterior portion of the capsule becomes adherent to the neck of the scapula posteriorly (Fig. 202). In addition, that part of the capsule lying across the glenoid becomes fixed to it by the contracture of the capsule and scar tissue formation in the glenoid fossa. In an old unreduced posterior dislocation the pathological changes tend to reverse themselves. The capsule then becomes adherent to the neck of the capsule anteriorly while that part of the capsule bow-stringing across the glenoid becomes somewhat contracted and bound down by scar tissue (Fig. 203).

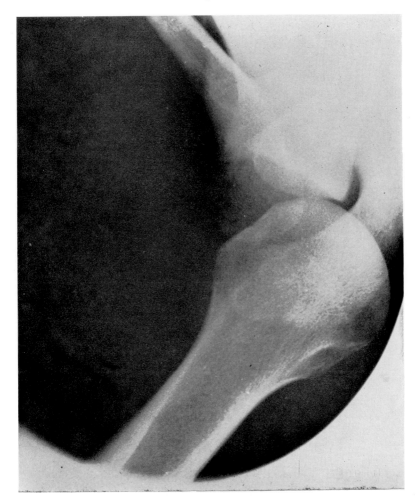

Figure 194. Posterior subluxation of the humeral head.

With a proper understanding of the pathological processes involved in old reduced anterior or posterior dislocations, one will not only be able to interpret the arthrographic findings but be able to correct these displacements by the operative procedure proposed by the author, namely, the "Stripping Operation." The operation is usually indicated in cases characterized by intractable pain from pressure upon the brachial plexus, occasionally from vascular changes or a combination of both of these factors. **Figure**

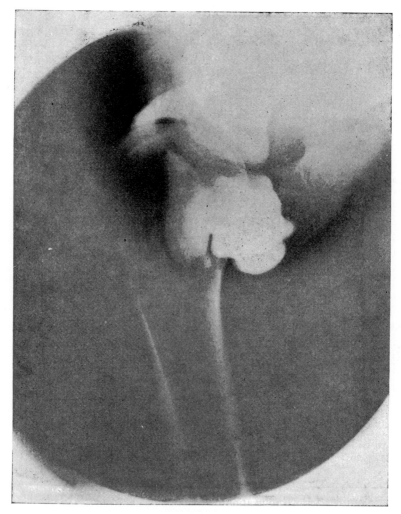

Figure 195. Axillary view of arthrogram. Observe the very redundant posterior capsule.

204 is an axillary view of an arthrogram of an unreduced anterior dislocation of the shoulder of seven weeks duration in a fifty-eight-year-old male. It demonstrates quite well the bow-stringing of the capsule across the glenoid. Closed reduction under general anesthesia was unsuccessful. The stripping operation was performed.

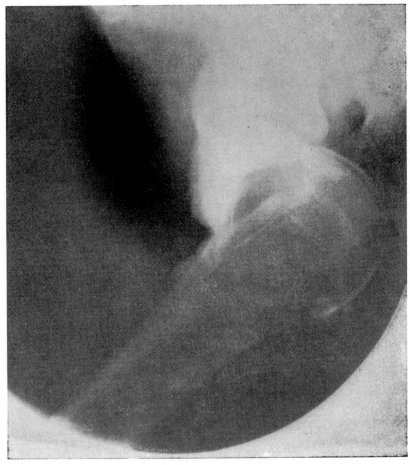

Figure 196. Head has subluxated backwards occupying the relaxed posterior capsular space. Most of the dye has been pushed forward filling the joint space opposite the glenoid.

Operative Technique for Reduction of Old Unreduced Dislocations

With the patient in the sitting position, under general anesthesia and the arm draped free, the superior or transacromial approach is used. This approach can be used for either old anterior or posterior unreduced dislocations. After the deltoid is retracted downward the capsule is exposed. It will be found stretched across

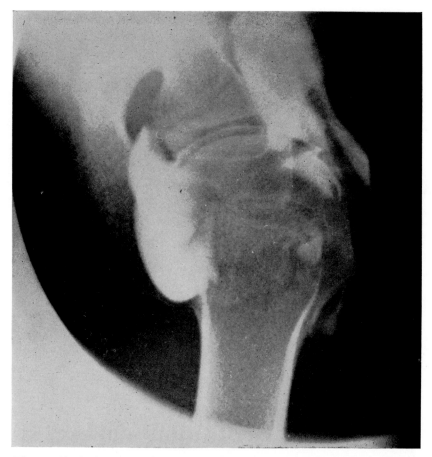

Figure 197. Arthrogram of right shoulder. Axillary view. Head in position. Note large subscapularis bursa anteriorly.

the glenoid fossa. In old unreduced anterior dislocations it may be necessary to strip the clavicular fibers of the deltoid off the anterior lateral surface of the clavicle. The capsule is opened by a longitudinal incision about 4.5 cm in length, just lateral to the insertion of the subscapularis tendon but past the bicipital groove. It is not necessary to cut the subscapularis muscle, thus avoiding injury to the axillary nerve as it passes backward below the subscapularis through the quadrilateral space to supply the deltoid and teres minor muscles. The attachments of the capsule

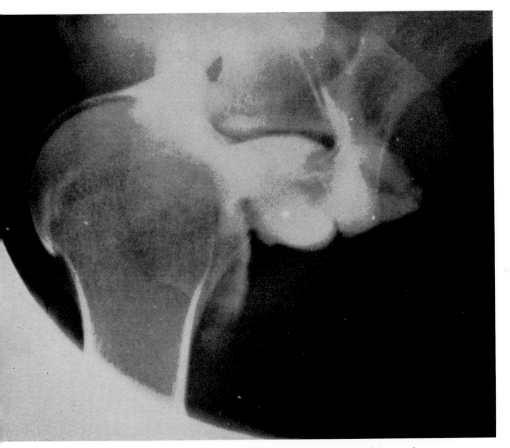

Figure 198. Arthrogram of right shoulder with the head subluxated posteriorly. The head fills the capsular space posteriorly. Observe the bowstringing of the capsule across the glenoid with the dye from the subscapularis bursa now lying in the space opposite the glenoid.

to the neck of the humerus are stripped away by the use of a sharp curved periosteal elevator or a gooseneck chisel and at times aided by the fingers. The stripping should be carried beyond the greater tuberosity and should include a portion of the neck medial to the lesser tuberosity. Subperiosteal separation of the tendons from the tuberosities does not interfere with their attachments to the musculotendinous cuff. At times, parts of the capsule that require stripping can be identified by palpation, with

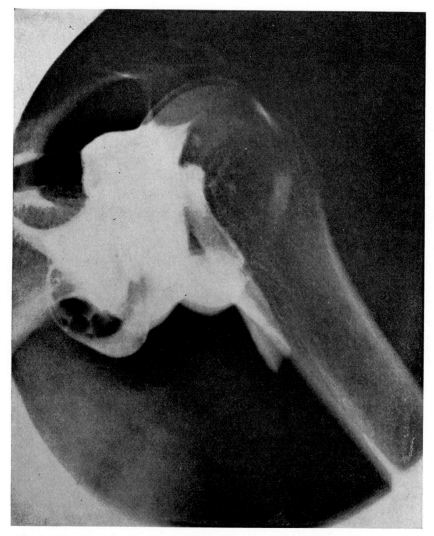

Figure 199. Arthrogram of the left shoulder which is subluxated posteriorly. Note the apparent medial displacement of the biceps sheath. Actually, this is due to the marked internal rotation of the humerus.

one or two fingers inserted through the opening in the capsule. In an old anterior dislocation every effort should be made to strip the adherent capsule from the posterior part of the neck of the scapula near the glenoid cavity, while in an old posterior dis-

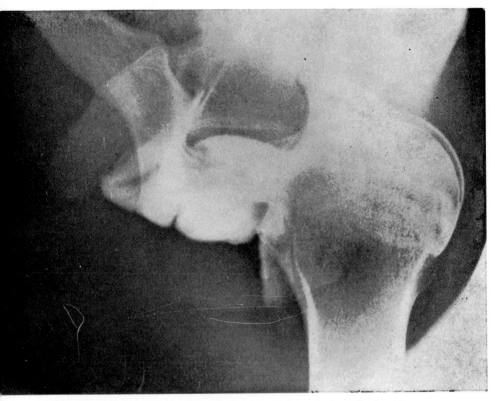

Figure 200. Axillary view of the arthrogram taken of the left shoulder seen in Figure 199 reveals the biceps sheath in its normal position. Again note the bow-stringing of the capsule across the glenoid.

location the capsule must be stripped away from the anterior surface of the scapular neck. After a thorough subperiosteal stripping the displaced head is sufficiently mobile to allow its reposition without undue tension. After the glenoid cavity is cleared of any scar tissue reduction is effected by pushing the head of the humerus laterally. This maneuver will disengage the head if it should be wedged up against the rim of the glenoid. The head is then easily placed in position opposite the glenoid cavity.

An important step in the operation is the holding of the head in position opposite the glenoid. This is done by the use of a long wood screw of vitallium, a pin or a heavy Kirschner wire,

NORMAL RELATIONSHIP

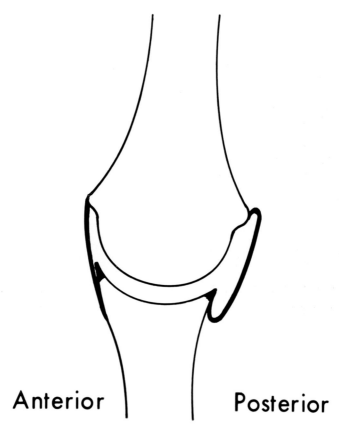

Anterior | Posterior

Figure 201. Outline of the normal relationship of the shoulder capsule as would be seen on the axillary view.

whichever is preferred by the surgeon. A small incision is made through the skin and other soft tissues directly lateral to the humeral head and the metal pin or screw is inserted through the head into the glenoid fossa. If the capsule can be closed or its

RELATIONSHIP
IN UNREDUCED
ANTERIOR DISLOCATION

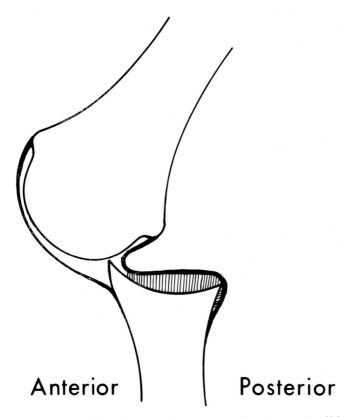

Anterior   Posterior

Figure 202. Relationship of the capsule in an unreduced anterior dislocation of the shoulder. The posterior part of the capsule becomes adherent to the scapular neck posteriorly. Scar tissue formation tends to fix the capsule across the glenoid.

edges sutured close to the head without tension, this is done; if not, no attempt is made to close or repair the capsule. It is believed that the remnants of the capsule will contract about the head during the healing process, and that, by the time the metal

RELATIONSHIP IN UNREDUCED POSTERIOR DISLOCATION

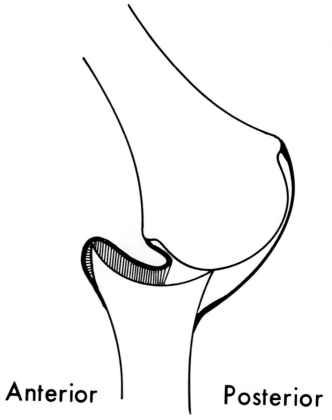

Anterior Posterior

Figure 203. In an unreduced posterior dislocation the capsule becomes adherent to the anterior surface of the scapular neck. That part of the capsule bow-stringing across the glenoid becomes adherent by scar tissue formation.

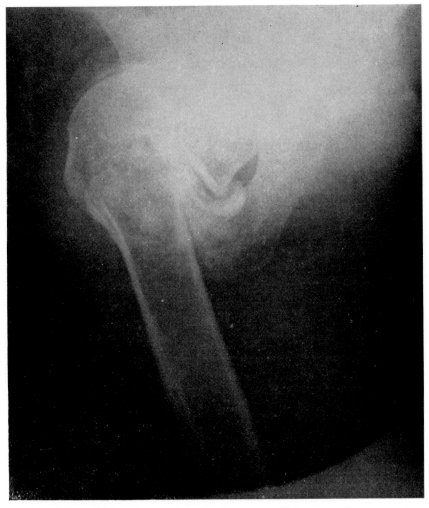

Figure 204. Arthrogram of an unreduced anterior dislocation of seven weeks duration. The axillary view demonstrates quite well the bow-stringing of the capsule across the glenoid. (Courtesy of *Surgical Clinics N.A.*, *43*:1671, December, 1963.)

fixation is removed, the head will be held firmly in proper positions.

Following closure of the wound the patient's arm is immobilized by his side by strapping or the application of a stockinette Velpeau in the position determined by the screw or pin. The

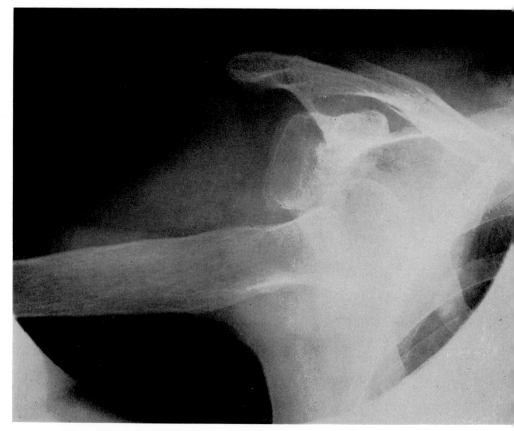

Figure 205. Subcoracoid dislocation of five weeks duration.

sutures are removed after ten days and the arm is placed in a sling. Forward flexion and backward extension of the shoulder are encouraged while the arm is supported in a sling. Three or four weeks after operation the small lateral operative scar is excised under local anesthesia and the metal screw or pin is removed. About a week later, when the wound of the second operation has healed, the sling is discarded, physical therapy is instituted and use of the arm is encouraged.

After this operation the patients have been relieved of their pain and the affected shoulders have regained useful function. If the arm could be actively abducted to an angle of 60 degrees at the glenohumeral joint the result was considered satisfactory. Patients that could actively abduct their arms to ninety degrees

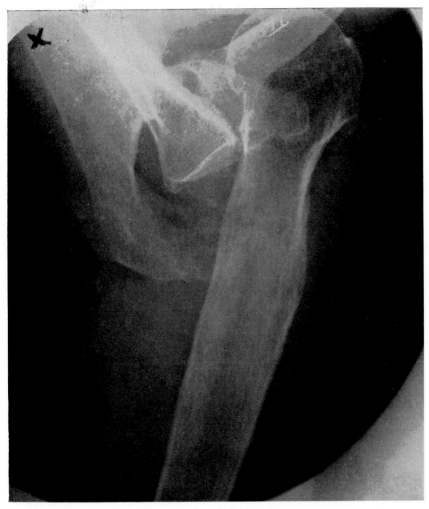

Figure 206. Axillary view reveals marked anterior displacement of the humeral head.

and some to 150 degrees were considered to have excellent results. No harmful changes due to the insertion of the metal fixation through the humeral head or glenoid have been noted in subsequent roentgenograms.

Illustrative Cases:

A male, age fifty-five years, was admitted to the hospital because of pain and numbness in his right hand. About five weeks prior to admission he fell and injured his right shoulder. He thought the pain would disappear but when he developed some numbness in his fingers which gradually involved his hand he finally sought medical advice. The roentgenograms revealed an anterior dislocation (Figs. 205, 206). On the anterior-posterior view the arthrogram showed dye escaping into the subdeltoid bursa and down along the under surface of the deltoid muscle (Fig. 207), indicative of a rupture associated with the dislocation, while the axillary view showed the capsule bowstringing across the glenoid (Fig. 208). The dye in the subdeltoid bursa tended to obscure the details of the glenoid anteriorly. Two attempts at closed reduction under general anesthesia were unsuccess-

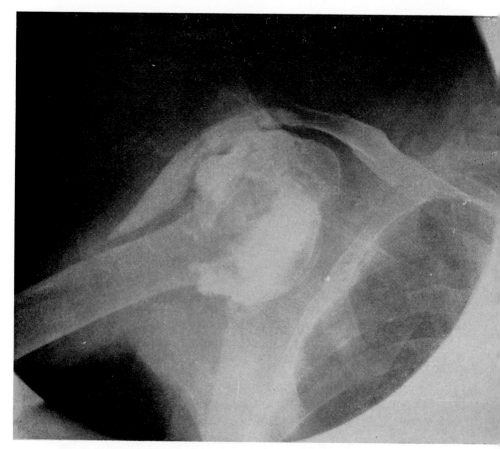

Figure 207. Arthrogram of the dislocated shoulder reveals dye extravasating into the subdeltoid bursa and along the plane of the deltoid. This was evidence of a rupture associated with the dislocation.

ful. An open reduction was done nine weeks after his injury. The capsule was stripped from the humeral head after extending the tear by incising the cuff proximally and distally. Reduction was then possible. We were able to suture the capsule after a screw was used to hold the head in position (Fig. 209). Three weeks later the screw was removed and pendulum exercises were carried out for one week with the arm in a sling. The humeral head remained in normal position (Fig. 210). Three months after operation the patient no longer had pain in his shoulder, and the numbness in his hand had disappeared. Abduction was 90 degrees (Fig. 211).

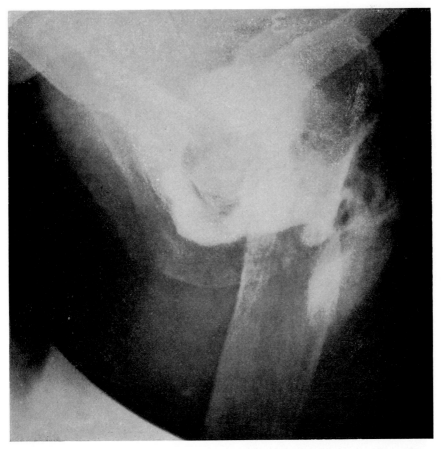

Figure 208. Axillary view shows the bow-stringing of the capsule across the glenoid although some of the dye in the subdeltoid bursa obscures the details of the joint anteriorly.

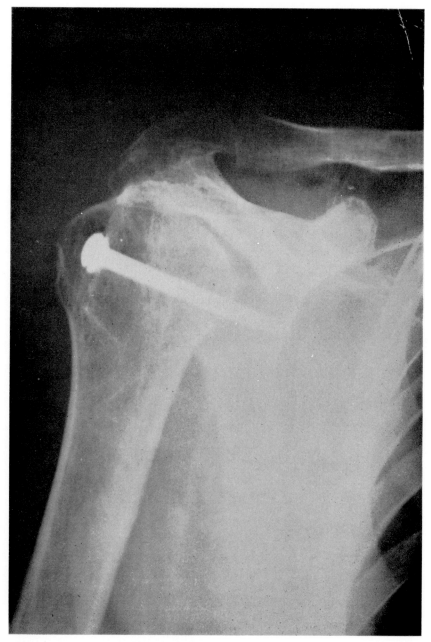

Figure 209. Humeral head is held in the position by a screw.

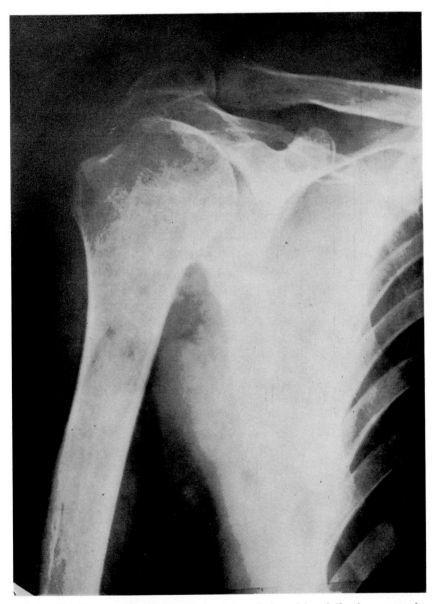

Figure 210. Humeral head remains in anatomical position following removal of the screw.

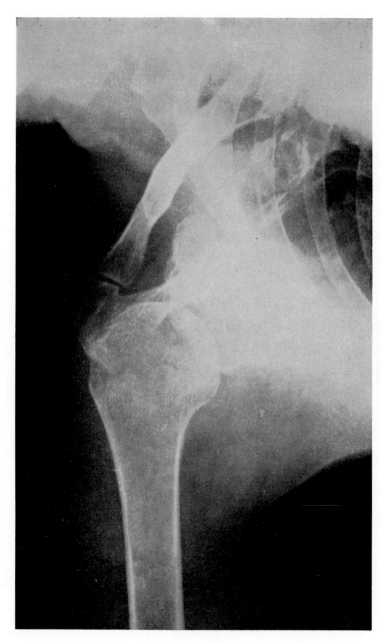

Figure 211. Abduction of ninety degrees three months after operation.

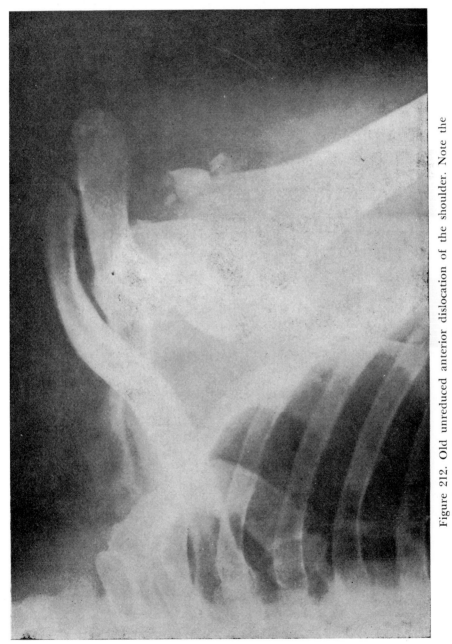

Figure 212. Old unreduced anterior dislocation of the shoulder. Note the comminution of the greater tuberosity.

A male, age forty-nine years, injured his left shoulder six weeks previously when he fell down a flight of stairs. He had a concussion syndrome and when he improved he came to the office for his persistent shoulder pain. Roentgenograms revealed an old dislocation with some comminution of the greater tuberosity (Fig. 212). An arthrogram revealed the dye pooling around the greater tuberosity fragment extending down to the upper part of the shaft of the humerus (Fig. 213). On the axillary view the dye was seen around the greater

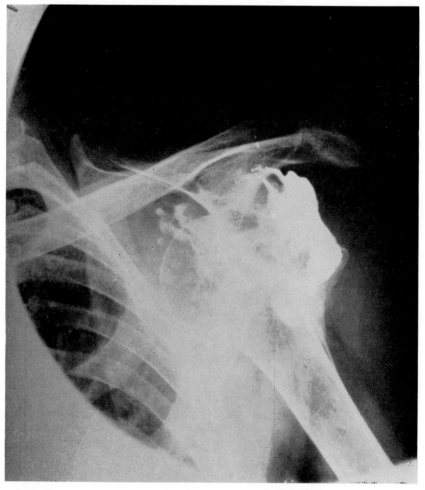

Figure 213. Arthrogram reveals pooling of much of the dye around the comminuted greater tuberosity fragment.

tuberosity, which was displaced posteriorly (Fig. 214). Close observation revealed the contrast medium obscuring the outline of the posterior part of the joint. When attempts at closed reduction failed the
stripping operation was performed eight weeks after injury. Following
this procedure the humeral head was placed in normal position and
held by a screw (Fig. 215). Three and one-half weeks later the screw
was removed. A sling was used for one week and then active motion
was encouraged. A film taken one week after removal of the screw
showed the head in the anatomical position (Fig. 216). Some of the
comminuted pieces of the greater tuberosity had been removed at

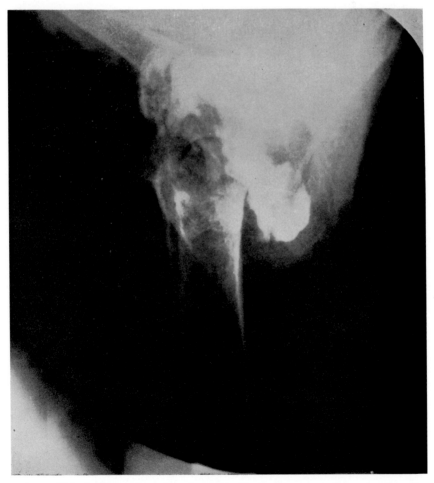

Figure 214. Axillary view of arthrogram. Dye again seen about the site of
the greater tuberosity fragments which are displaced posteriorly.

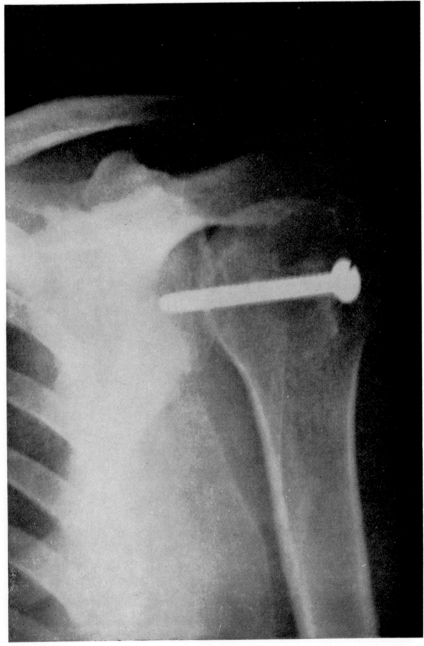

Figure 215. After reduction of the dislocation by the stripping operation. Screw holds the head in good position.

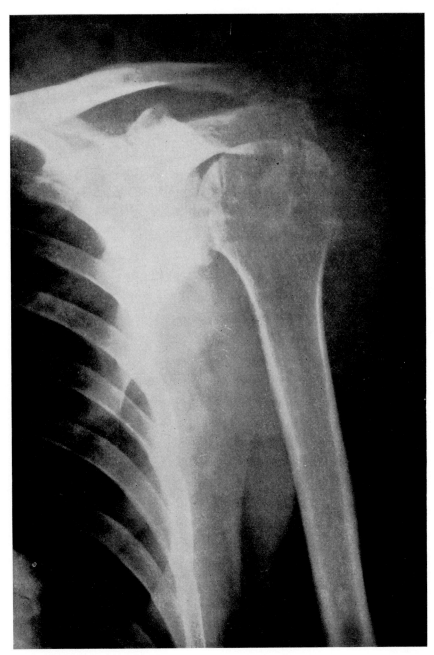

Figure 216. Appearance of shoulder one week after removal of the screw.

operation. After two months abduction was 100 degrees and the patient was relieved of most of his pain.

A male, aged thirty-six years, fell and injured his right shoulder two and one-half months prior to his admission to the hospital. He complained of constant pain in his shoulder with very little use of his

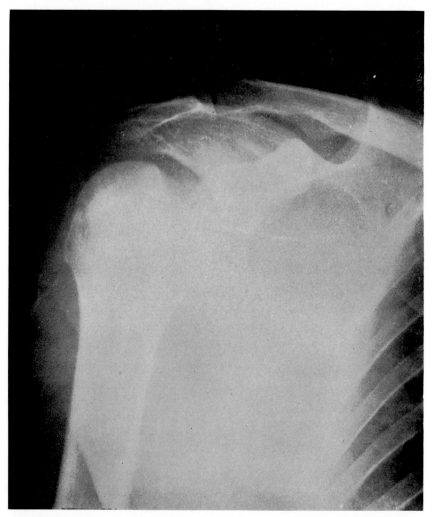

Figure 217. Old unreduced posterior dislocation of the shoulder. A-P view taken about ten weeks after injury. (Courtesy of *Surgical Clinics N.A., 43*:1671, December, 1963.)

arm. Roentgenograms revealed an old unreduced posterior dislocation of the shoulder (Figs. 217, 218). On the axillary view a notch
was seen in the humeral head as well as a fracture of the lesser tuberosity. *If a fracture of the lesser tuberosity is ever seen on the anterior-
posterior view one should always suspect a posterior dislocation.* When

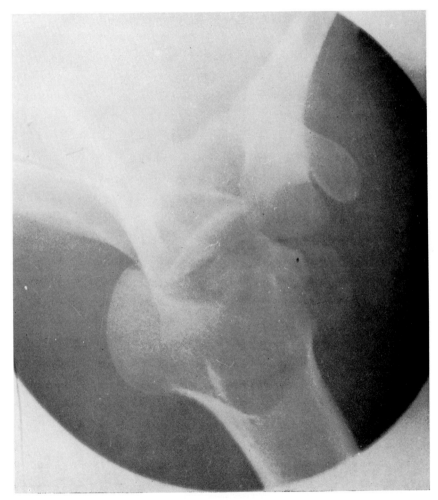

Figure 218. Axillary view reveals a notch in the humeral head following impingement against the posterior rim of the glenoid. A fracture of the lesser
tuberosity is barely discernible. (Courtesy of *Surgical Clinics N.A., 43*:1671,
December, 1963.)

closed reduction failed, an open operation was performed three months after injury. Using the superior approach the capsule was incised and stripped from the upper humerus and anterior part of the neck of the scapula. The dislocated head was reduced without difficulty and held in position by the insertion of a stout pin (Fig. 219). The axillary

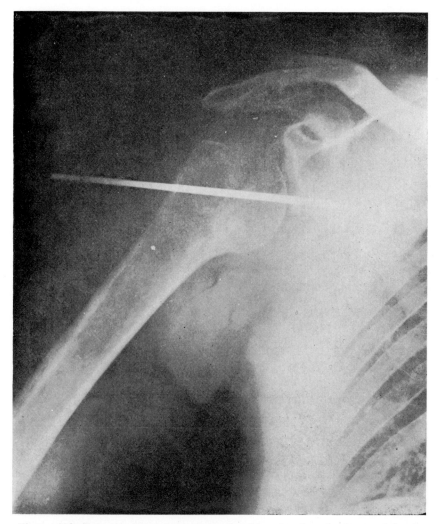

Figure 219. Post-operative view of the shoulder showing the humeral head held in position by a stout pin. (Courtesy of *Surgical Clinics of N.A.*, *43*:1671, December, 1963.)

view revealed the head in good position (Fig. 220). The pin was removed after three and one-half weeks and the arm placed in a sling for one week. After eight weeks the patient could abduct to 75 degrees and his pain was minimal. The appearance of the humeral head was good and on the axillary view the notch in the head appears to have disappeared (Figs. 221, 222). The patient reached maximum abduction of 95 degrees four months after operation.

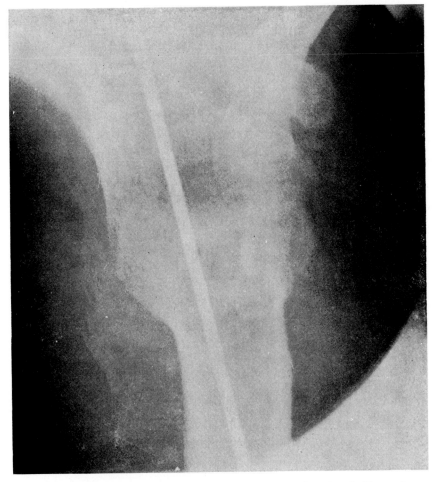

Figure 220. Excellent position of the head held by the pin. Axillary view. (Courtesy of *Surgical Clinics of N.A., 43*:1671, December, 1963.)

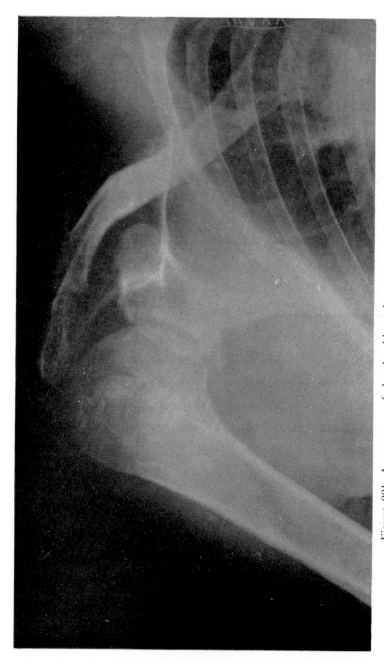

Figure 221. Appearance of the shoulder taken two months after operation. Note good contour of the humeral head. (Courtesy of *Surgical Clinics N.A.*, *43*:1071, December, 1963.)

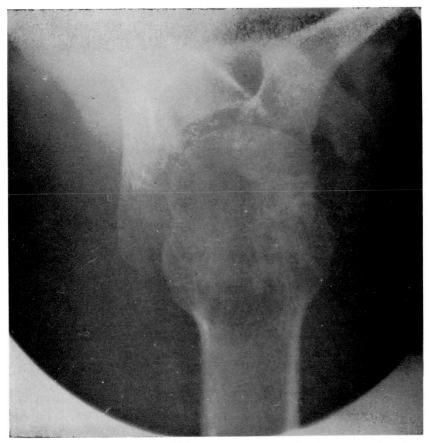

Figure 222. The axillary view shows the head in good position. Note that the compression notch in the head is hardly visible. (Courtesy of *Surgical Clinics N.A., 43:*1671, December, 1963.)

The "stripping operation" described for old unreduced dislocations of the shoulder offers the following advantages:

1. The superior or sabre cut approach can be used for either old anterior or posterior unreduced dislocations.
2. The reduction is facilitated by opening the joint capsule and stripping it from the humeral head and anatomical neck.
3. The danger of injuring the axillary nerve is minimized by avoiding division of the subscapularis.

4. The relationship of the tendons to the musculotendinous cuff is undisturbed.
5. Postoperative redislocation is prevented by internal fixation with a transfixing screw, a stout pin or a small Knowles pin.
6. Surgical repair of the joint capsule is not essential. If the cuff cannot be sutured without tension, it can be allowed to heal and contract about the humeral head.
7. Stiffness of the shoulder joint is minimized by mobilization after early removal of the transfixing screw or pin.

FRACTURES OF THE SURGICAL NECK OF THE HUMERUS

F RACTURES OF THE SURGICAL NECK of the humerus, occasionally accompanied by a fracture of the greater tuberosity, have left many patients with some pain and significant limitation of motion in the shoulder. If the roentgenograms show satisfactory position of the fracture with good union, then the explanation for this restriction of motion becomes even more perplexing. Some patients have been thought to have an adhesive capsulitis but a manipulation under general anesthesia has resulted in little, if any, improvement in shoulder motion or diminution of pain.

Arthrography has been helpful in determining the cause of this condition. The capsule becomes adherent to the anatomical neck, particularly at the anterior-superior part of the neck. The serrations that are normally seen where the capsule is attached to the anatomical neck are obliterated and, in some instances, the biceps tendon is bound down in the groove. The lesion, in a sense, is similar to an adhesive capsulitis, but in such cases the dependent fold is always visualized on the arthrograms, while in the cases of adhesive capsulitis, the dependent axillary fold is obliterated. Exercises or manipulations seldom help these patients and, if the restriction of motion and pain are marked, then an open operation is indicated.

The exposure of the shoulder is usually made through the anterior axillary approach unless there are other abnormalities visualized on the arthrograms, such as a binding down of the biceps tendon or a tear of the rotator cuff. The superior-anterior approach through the delto-pectoral groove, or the acromioclavicular arthroplasty as advocated by Bateman can then be used.

The rotator cuff is incised superiorly between the aponeurosis of the external and internal rotators of the shoulder just lateral to the bicipital groove. After opening the capsule, the area of adherence to the anatomical neck can be located and, using a joker or a small periosteal elevator, the adherent capsule can be separated from the articular surface of the humeral head down

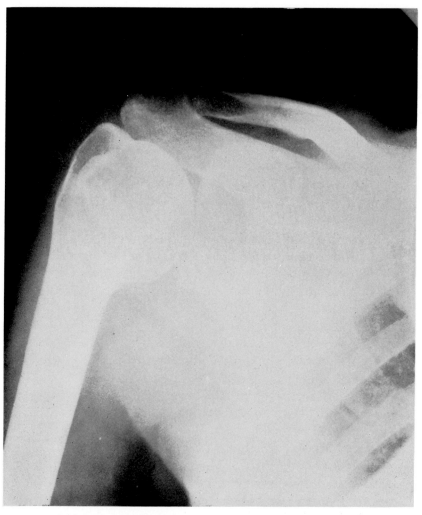

Figure 223. Fracture of the surgical neck shows good healing after eighteen months. Position is satisfactory.

to the anatomical neck. The improvement in motion is tested by gentle movements of the arm in all directions. If the biceps sheath reveals a definite tenosynovitis the tendon can be resected and the distal portion fixed in the bicipital groove. If the capsule has been opened through the site of tear, it is then repaired. Following closure of the capsule early motion is encouraged

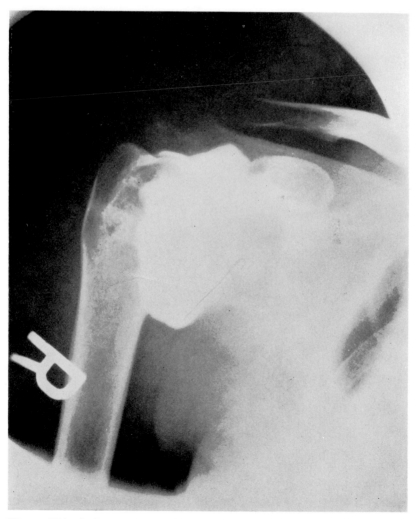

Figure 224. Arthrogram reveals lack of filling of the capsule near the anatomical neck superiorly due to a binding down of the capsule at this site.

after the first postoperative day with the arm in a sling. If there has been a tear of the cuff or the biceps tendon has been resected, the shoulder should be immobilized for three weeks. It is discarded after the sutures have been removed.

Case Reports:

Y. F., a white female, aged forty-nine years, was seen ten days after a fall on the beach. She had sustained a fracture of the surgical neck and greater tuberosity of the right humerus. A hanging cast had been applied. Since the roentgenograms revealed satisfactory position of the fragments the hanging cast was allowed to remain on the arm for one month. Pendulum exercises were given the patient following removal of the cast. A sling was used to support the arm for another

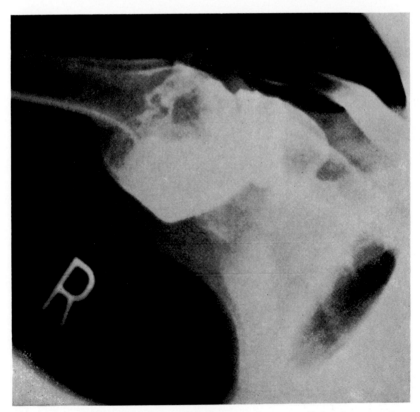

Figure 225. Arthrogram taken with the arm in some abduction reveals a definite paucity of dye around the anatomical neck superiorly.

week. After discarding the sling physical therapy and exercises were instituted. When seen eighteen months later this patient complained of pain and limitation of motion. Active abduction was 145 degrees. Roentgenograms taken of the right shoulder revealed the fractures to be well healed in good position (Fig. 223). Arthrograms revealed a binding down of the capsule near the upper part of the anatomical neck which prevented entrance of the dye at that site (Fig. 224). With the arm in abduction less dye is seen penetrating or distending the capsule (Fig. 225). Following operative stripping of the adherent capsule from the articular surface of the humeral head down to the anatomical neck, the patient was able to abduct the arm painlessly to 175 degrees after three months.

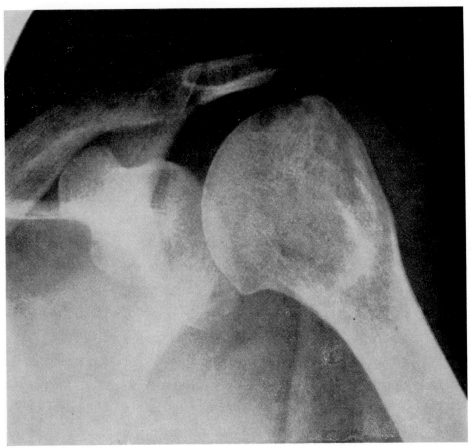

Figure 226. Healed fractures of the greater tuberosity and surgical neck noted fourteen months after injury.

E. W., a male, forty-two years of age, was seen fourteen months after he fell from a scaffold injuring his left shoulder and left foot. He had sustained a fracture of the surgical neck of the left humerus and greater tuberosity. No fractures of the left foot were seen on the roentgenograms of the foot. The left arm had been placed in a sling which he wore for six weeks. Active use and exercises were prescribed for the patient. When his shoulder pain continued with limitation of motion he was referred to me for care. Active abduction of the shoulder was one hundred degrees, external rotation thirty degrees, and upon internal rotation the left hand touched only two inches above the belt line.

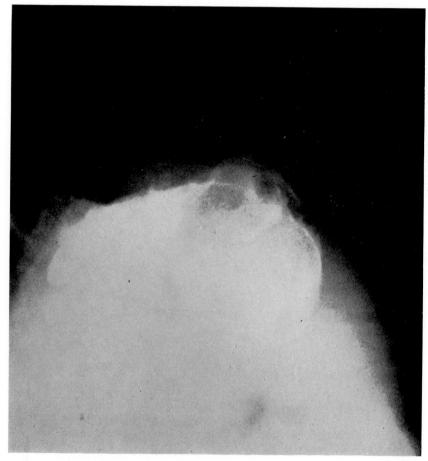

Figure 227. Bicipital groove view reveals a bony bridge over the bicipital groove extending from the lesser tuberosity close to the greater tuberosity.

Roentgenograms taken fourteen months after injury revealed a healed fracture of the greater tuberosity and surgical neck of the humerus (Fig. 226) apparently in good position. The axillary view showed some excess bone formation about the lesser tuberosity, while the bicipital groove view revealed what appeared to be a bony bridge over the groove extending from the lesser tuberosity close to the greater tuberosity (Fig. 227).

The arthrograms showed no rupture but an adherence of the capsule near the upper part of the anatomical neck (Fig. 228). A good dependent axillary fold was visualized but no dye was seen filling the biceps sheath. With the arm abducted to 90 degrees, very little dye had extravasated into the biceps sheath or the upper lateral part of the

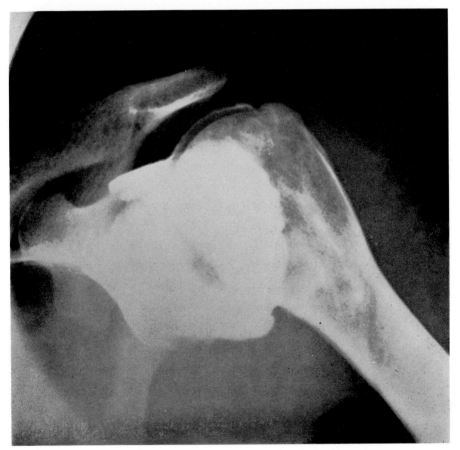

Figure 228. Arthrogram demonstrates lack of filling of the joint superiorly near the anatomical neck. Biceps sheath not visualized.

capsule (Fig. 229). On the axillary view of the arthrogram the biceps sheath did not take any dye and there was a lack of filling of the capsule at the anterior part of its attachment to the anatomical neck (Fig. 230).

At operation using the superior-anterior approach the upper part of the capsule was stripped from the head near the anatomical neck. The bridge of bone was removed from the lesser tuberosity and the biceps sheath and tendon were unroofed. The sheath was thickened and inflammed. It was dissected out, the intraarticular portion of the tendon was resected, and the distal portion fixed in the bicipital groove, after

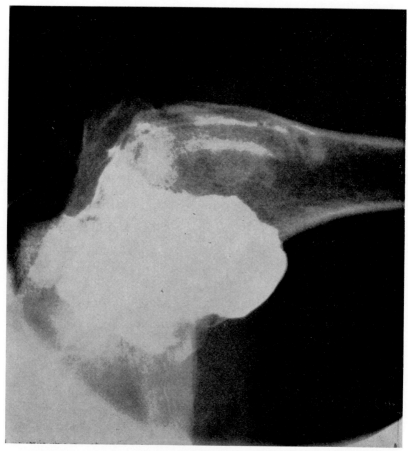

Figure 229. With the arm abducted to ninety degrees very little dye is present about the anatomical neck superiorly. Biceps sheath is outlined by some dye in the sheath.

deepening and roughening the groove. Following wound closure a
stockinette Velpeau dressing was applied. After three weeks it was removed and a sling was used. It was discarded after one week and active
use and exercises were encouraged. After four months this patient
could abduct his left arm to 170 degrees and his discomfort was minimal.

K. B., a female, sixty-five years of age, fell forward on a step and
injured her right shoulder eleven months prior to the time I saw her.
She sustained a fracture of the surgical neck and greater tuberosity of
the humerus. The arm was immobilized in a Velpeau dressing for a
period of five weeks. She received physical therapy and exercises after
the Velpeau dressing was discharged.

Her pain and limitation of motion continued with very little im-

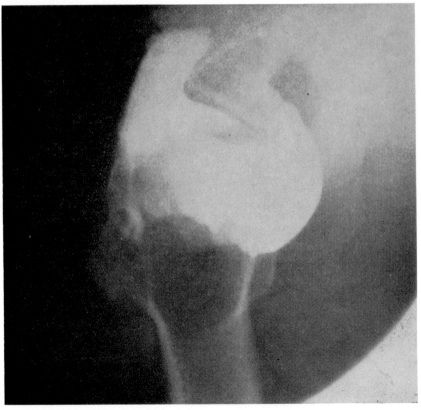

Figure 230. Axillary view reveals lack of filling of the capsule at its attachment to the anatomical neck anteriorly.

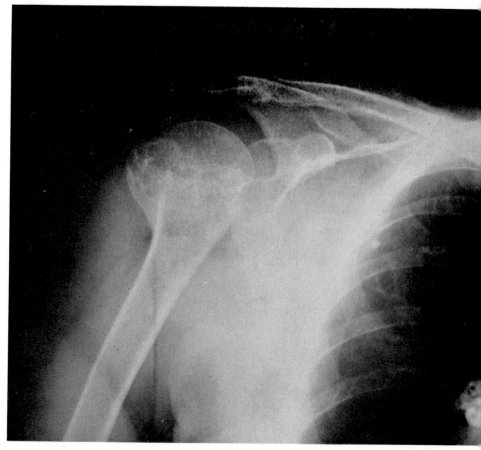

Figure 231. Roentgenogram taken eleven months after an injury reveals a healed fracture of the greater tuberosity and surgical neck.

provement after six months of therapy. At the time of my examination active abduction was 85 degrees. Upon internal rotation the right hand could only reach three inches above the belt line. Roentgenograms taken at that time revealed a healed fracture of the greater tuberosity and surgical neck on the internal rotation view (Fig. 231) while on the external rotation view the greater tuberosity fragment was displaced upward.

The arthrogram revealed a lack of filling by the dye at the upper part of the anatomical neck. The serrations of the capsule at its attachment to the anatomical neck superiorly had been obliterated (Fig. 232). With the arm in some abduction there was still a lack of filling with the dye of the capsule at its attachment to the anatomical neck superiorly (Fig. 233).

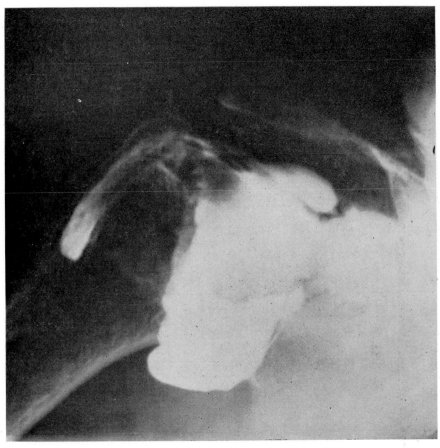

Figure 232. Arthrogram shows absence of the serrations of the capsule at its attachment to the anatomical neck superiorly as well as incomplete filling by the dye at that site.

At operation, which was performed one year after her accident, an acromioplasty was done including a section of the coracoacromial ligament. The displaced greater tuberosity fragment was discarded and the cuff fixed to the upper part of the humerus near the surgical neck with silk sutures passed through drill holes. The capsule was stripped from the upper part of the humeral head down to the anatomical neck. After closure the arm was immobilized in a stockinette Velpeau dressing for a period of three weeks. After removal of the dressing a sling was used for one week, with the patient performing pendulum exercises during that time. After the sling was discarded full use and exercise were encouraged. The pain decreased as the motion of her

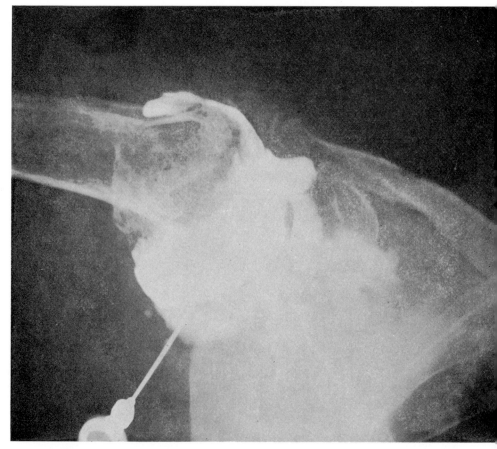

Figure 233. Arthrogram taken with the arm in ninety degrees of abduction. There is still a lack of filling by the dye at the upper part of the humeral head near the anatomical neck.

shoulder increased. After six months active abduction was 135 degrees and her pain was minimal.

The above described cases demonstrate how pain and limitation of motion resulting from a fracture of the surgical neck with or without a fracture of the greater tuberosity can be relieved by stripping the adherent capsule from the humeral head down to the anatomical neck, particularly at the anterior-superior portion of the neck, where the pathologic process generally occurs.

Chapter Eight

INTERESTING CASES

I N THIS CHAPTER, the author would like to share with the reader, some interesting cases in which arthrography was of value in arriving at the diagnosis:

A. H., male, aged twenty-three years, was seen because of inability to abduct his left shoulder. He had an acromionectomy performed eighteen months previously for a recurrent dislocation of the shoulder. A Nicola procedure had been done two years before but this had failed. After this second operation he could not actively abduct his arm although upon passive abduction the arm could be elevated to 170 degrees. A routine A-P roentgenogram revealed that the acromion had been resected completely (Fig. 234). With the arm held in some abduction, wire sutures could be visualized in the soft tissues (Fig. 235). An arthrogram taken with the arm at the side revealed a lack of filling of the capsule superiorly (Fig. 236) but with the arm in abduction, dye was seen extravasating superiorly under the deltoid muscle (Fig. 237). At operation two conditions were found to account for this patient's difficulty. The capsule had been opened to perform the Nicola procedure but for some unexplained reason it had not been closed as no suture material could be found about the cuff edges. In addition, the middle fibers of the trapezius muscle which had been detached from the medial margin of the acromion after the removal of this bone segment had not been sutured to the central fibers of the deltoid. After closing the rotator cuff and anchoring the deltoid to the trapezius the appearance of the shoulder was not only enhanced but the patient obtained a good functioning arm.

J. C., male, fifty-two years, gave a history of someone pulling severely on his left arm about two years prior to the time he was first seen. He complained of a "giving way" feeling in his shoulder but pain was minimal. Upon examination there was a depression felt between the acromion and the humeral head. Motions of the shoulder were good although he had this feeling of insecurity when the arm was elevated to 170 degrees of abduction. Roentgenograms revealed downward subluxation of the humeral head (Fig. 238). The axillary view was

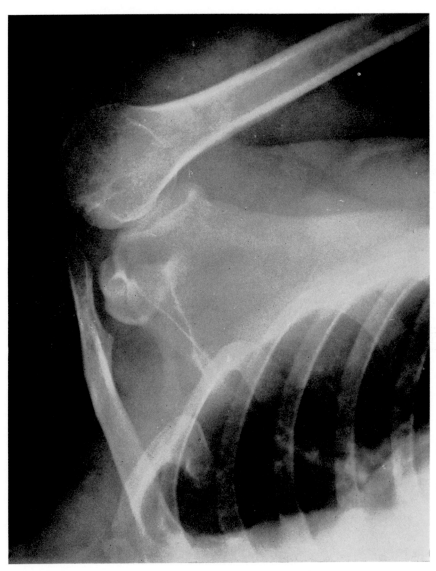

Figure 234. X-rays show that the acromion has been resected. Upward riding of the humeral head is also seen.

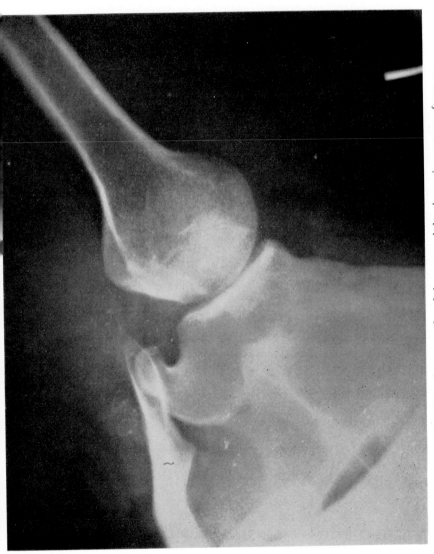

Figure 235. With the arm placed in some abduction wire sutures from a previous operation are visible.

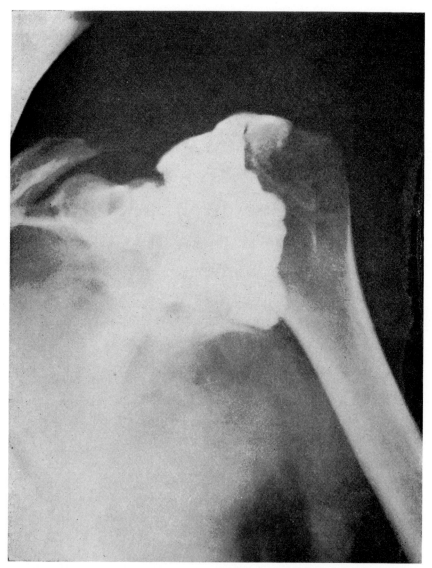

Figure 236. On the arthrogram there is incomplete filling by the dye superiorly near the anatomical neck.

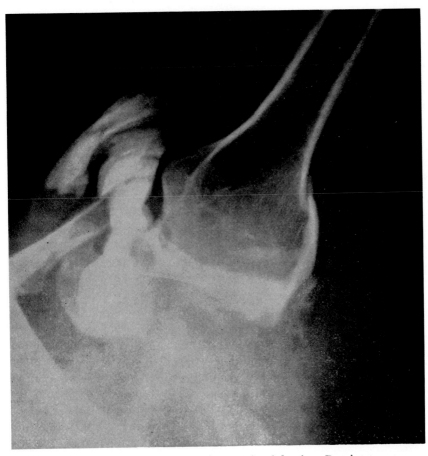

Figure 237. Arthrogram taken with the arm in abduction. Dye is seen escaping superiorly under the deltoid.

normal in appearance. Arthrograms revealed a stretching of the capsule near the glenoid with some escape of dye superiorly (Fig. 239). The arthrogram taken in the axillary view again showed the head in a normal position (Fig. 240). This is understandable since the head is displaced downward in line with the glenoid and not anteriorly or posteriorly in relation to the glenoid. At operation a small tear of the cuff was repaired, after fixing the edges of the capsule to the upper margins of the glenoid, anteriorly and posteriorly in the same manner as one would do a Bankart repair. Following immobilization of the arm for a period of three weeks, and a sling for one week, active use

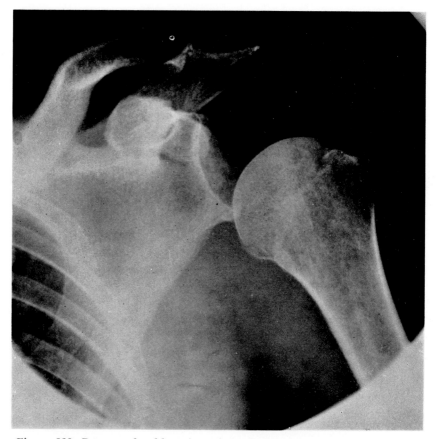

Figure 238. Downward subluxation of the humeral head easily seen on a routine A-P view.

and exercise was encouraged. The "giving way" feeling had disappeared.

M. H., male, eighteen years of age, was seen because of a feeling of the arm going out of joint. There was no history of an injury and the patient had very little pain during these episodes. Motions of the left shoulder were excellent. An X-ray revealed a loose body present in the axillary space (Fig. 241). An arthrogram showed the loose body to be in the joint lying within the dependent axillary fold (Fig. 242). When the loose body was removed the patient's symptoms disappeared.

R. H., female, fifty-six years, was seen because of an acute painful shoulder. The onset of pain was sudden and abduction was quite

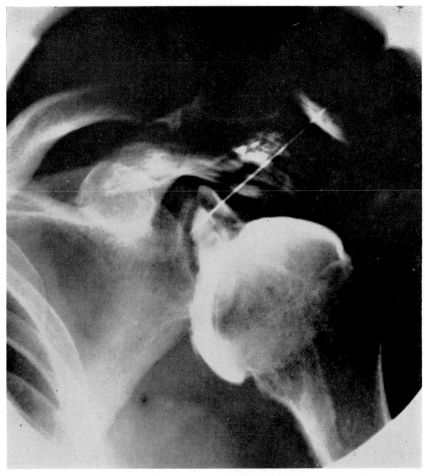

Figure 239. Arthrogram reveals a stretching of the capsule near the glenoid with some escape of the dye superiorly. Needle still in the joint.

painful. Tenderness was elicited just behind the greater tuberosity. X-rays revealed an area of calcification just above the greater tuberosity (Fig. 243). To prove that these sites of calcification in the substance of the tendon were extraarticular arthrography was performed and the arthrogram revealed an intact cuff with no communication between the joint and calcified area (Fig. 244).

T. R., male, twenty-eight years, first dislocated his right shoulder four years prior to the time I saw him. He had lifted a heavy weight

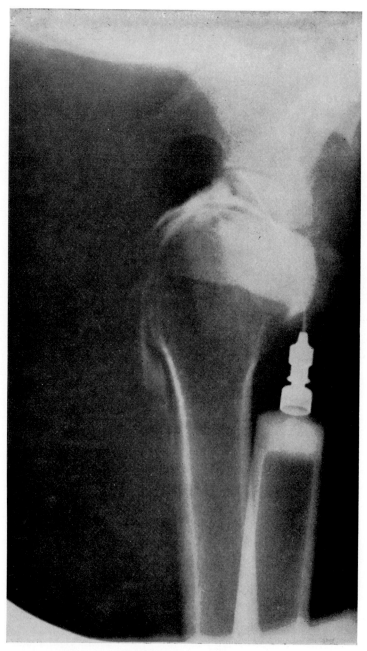

Figure 240. Axillary view of arthrogram shows the humeral head in good position. Dye still being instilled in the joint.

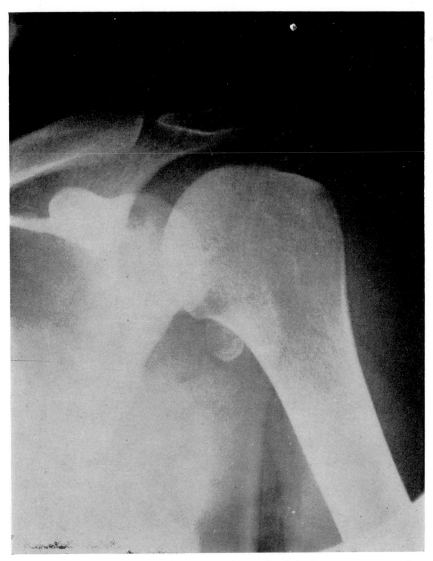

Figure 241. Loose body seen just below the neck of the humerus apparently within the joint space.

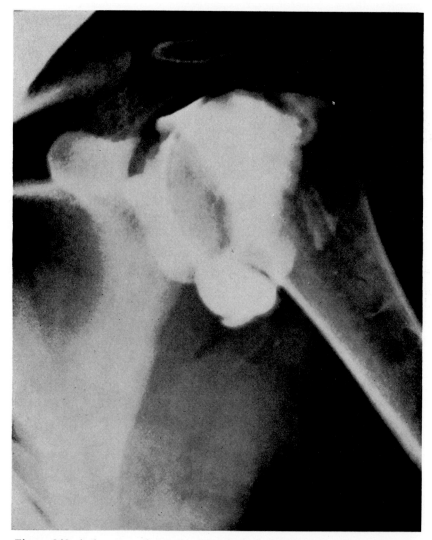

Figure 242. Arthrogram shows the loose body in the joint at the dependent axillary fold.

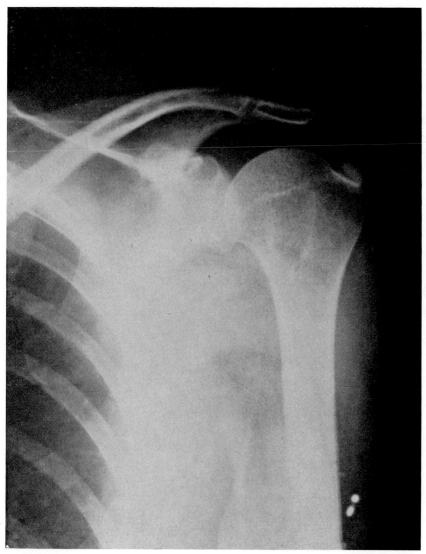

Figure 243. Area of calcification seen in the substance of the supraspinatus tendon.

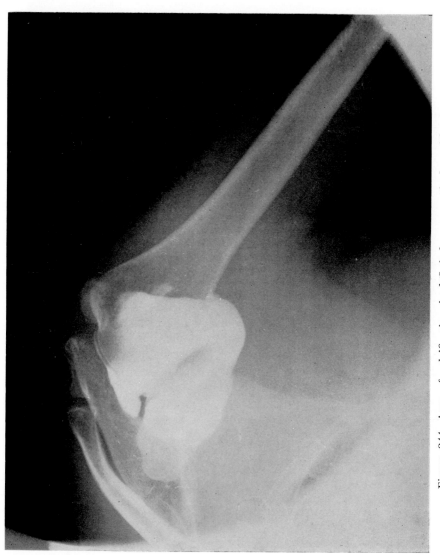

Figure 244. Area of calcification is definitely extra-articular with no communication between the joint and area of calcification.

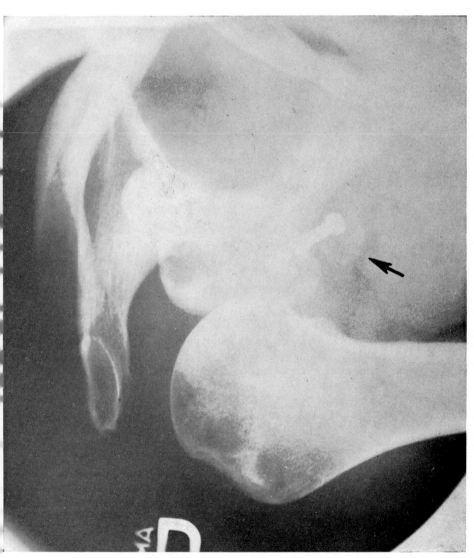

Figure 245. An area of calcification is seen about the screw head.

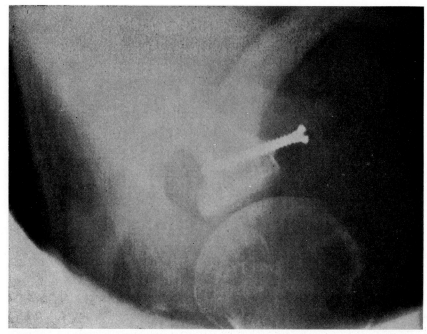

Figure 246. Axillary view shows that part of the coracoid has been resected and fixed by the screw into the neck of the scapula anteriorly.

and it fell on his shoulder causing a dislocation. The shoulder was reduced under general anesthesia and immobilized for three weeks. After frequent recurrences, especially when playing tennis, a Bristow procedure was done three years later. After a year he had no recurrences but he had pain anteriorly over the joint. An X-ray revealed that a resection of the tip of the coracoid process had been performed with fixation of the bone fragment into the neck of the scapula with a screw. An area of calcification was seen around the head of the screw (Figs. 245–246). Arthrograms showed the cuff intact (Fig. 247) but a slight displacement of the capsule from the neck of the scapula anteriorly on the axillary view (Fig. 248). With removal of the screw and roughening the neck of the scapula anteriorly followed by a Putti-Platt type of repair the pain was relieved.

A twenty-two-year-old male was seen in consultation because of pain and a "giving way" feeling in his left shoulder which had a gradual onset about six months previously. The discomfort and feeling had increased in the past month. He gave no history of an injury. The

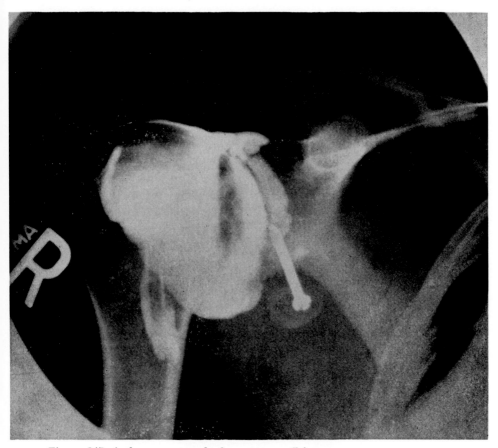

Figure 247. Arthrogram reveals the rotator cuff intact.

clinical findings revealed excellent range of motion in the shoulder with no points of tenderness. The roentgenograms revealed the presence of multiple loose bodies (Fig. 249). An arthrogram revealed the bodies to be contained within the joint capsule (Fig. 250). At operation many loose bodies of various sizes were removed (Fig. 251). His postoperative recovery was uneventful. He obtained good range of motion in the shoulder with relief from his complaints.

D. S., a fifty-nine-year-old male, fell off a scaffold injuring his right shoulder four months prior to the time that he was seen by me. He had a complete rupture of the rotator cuff which was repaired one week later by another orthopedic surgeon. The superior approach was used.

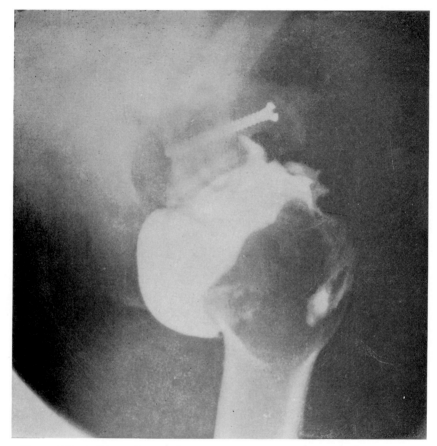

Figure 248. Axillary view of the arthrogram shows a slight displacement of the capsule from the scapular neck anteriorly.

Intensive physical therapy and exercises were outlined for him after his Velpeau dressing was discarded about three weeks following his surgery. Examination revealed active abduction to be 25 degrees and upon internal rotation he could only reach his buttock. Arthrography was performed ten days later or four and one-half months after surgery. The roentgenograms revealed extensive calcification about the humeral head, extending from the resected end of the acromion to below the greater tuberosity (Fig. 252). The axillary view showed spur formation from the acromion with some calcification distal to the spur-ring (Fig. 253). The arthrograms reveal the areas of calcification to be extraarticular with the possibility of some leakage of the dye superiorly

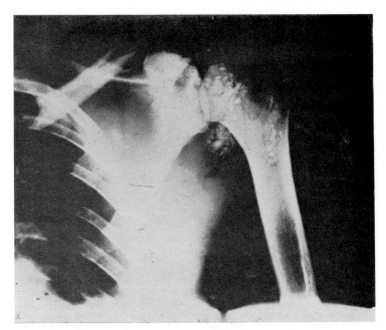

Figure 249. Multiple loose bodies seen on routine X-ray examination.

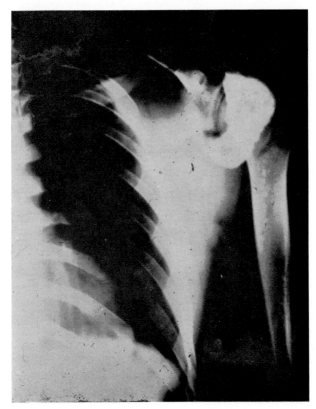

Figure 250. An arthrogram reveals the loose bodies to be present within the joint cavity.

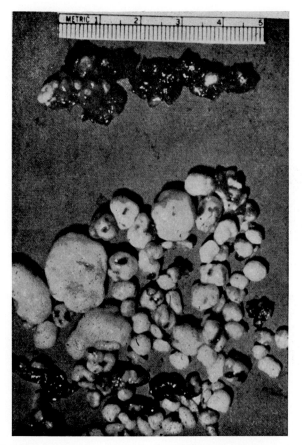

Figure 251. Note various sizes of the loose bodies removed from the shoulder joint.

(Fig. 254). The arthrogram taken in the axillary view also reveals the calcification to be outside of the joint capsule (Fig. 255). The bicipital groove view of the arthrogram again demonstrated the calcified mass to be lateral to the greater tuberosity (Fig. 256).

A sixty-six-year-old male had his right shoulder operated upon for a rupture of the rotator cuff four months after developing pain in his right shoulder without any history of an injury. The superior approach was used. Although he was relieved of much of his pain following the surgery he still had some discomfort in the shoulder with limitation of motion. The discomfort and restriction of motion persisted despite physical therapy and exercises. Three years after operation active ab-

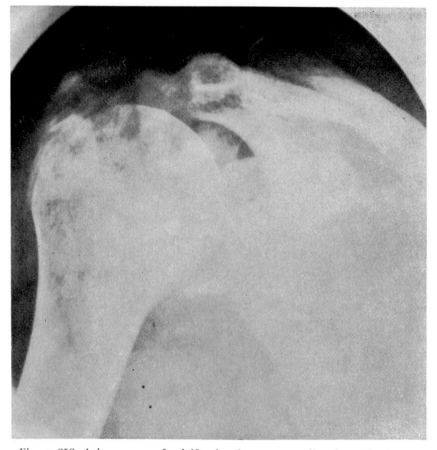

Figure 252. A large mass of calcification is seen extending from the lateral edge of the resected acromion to below the greater tuberosity.

duction was 120 degrees. A roentgenogram taken at that time revealed an area of calcification which appeared to follow the outline of the deltoid muscle (Fig. 257).

Although periarticular calcification of the shoulder was reported by me about twenty years ago as a rare complication of dislocation of the shoulder and also mentioned briefly by Watson-Jones, I have now seen five cases of periarticular calcification as a complication following arthrotomy of the shoulder using the superior or sabre cut approach. This may be a form of myositis

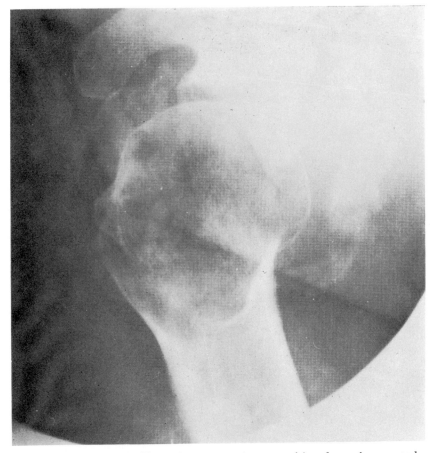

Figure 253. On the axillary view a spur is seen arising from the resected end of the acromion with some calcification distal to the spur.

ossificans but it seems to differ in two respects; it does not absorb and the patient has more pain in the joint. It follows the pattern of those cases of periarticular calcification that occur after a shoulder dislocation. No form of therapy has yet been found which promotes absorption of the calcification and permits restoration of full motion in the shoulder with subsequent decrease in pain.

A recent study of heterotopic ossification was reported by Nakaseko. His conclusions were based on investigations of clini-

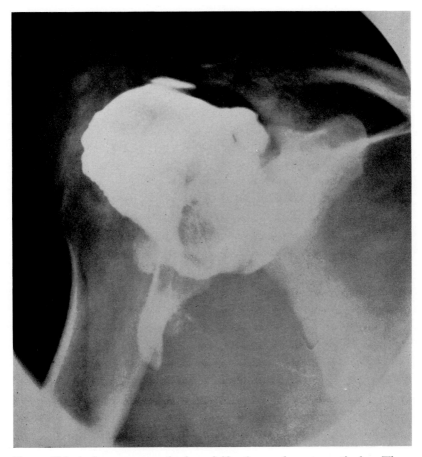

Figure 254. Arthrogram reveals the calcification to be extra-articular. There appears to be some leakage of dye superiorly.

cal material covering arterio-phlebographic, histological and biochemical findings on twenty-three cases of heterotopic ossification. It was established that blood stasis containing large amounts of organic and inorganic components was one of the important factors in the formation of the ossification. He felt that continuous local irrigation with ethylene-diamine-tetra-acetic acid (EDTA) and prednisolone acetate solution would appear to be the more effective method of preventing heterotopic ossification.

M. D., a male, fifty-six years of age, was seen seven weeks after his injury. He was loading a roller on a tractor trailer when he caught

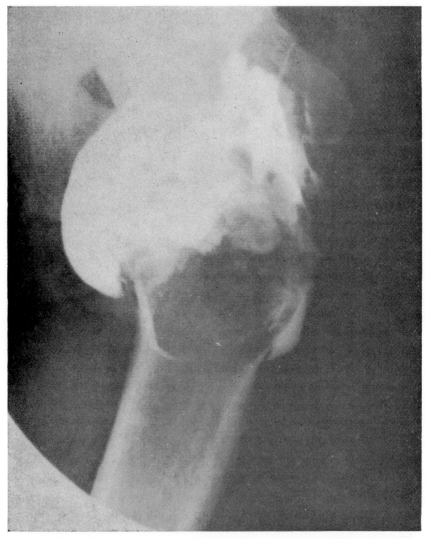

Figure 255. Axillary view of the arthrogram. The area of calcification is again seen extra-articular.

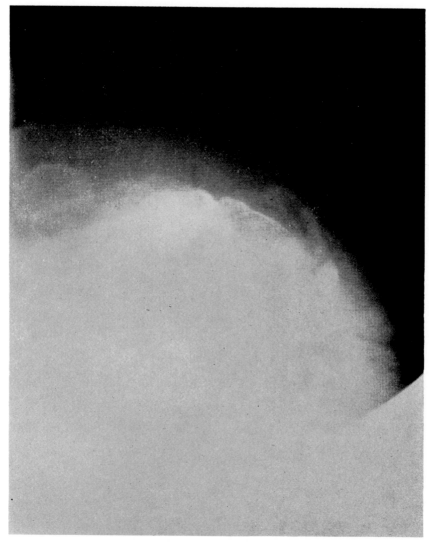

Figure 256. Bicipital groove view of the arthrogram. Note the area of calcification overlying the greater tuberosity.

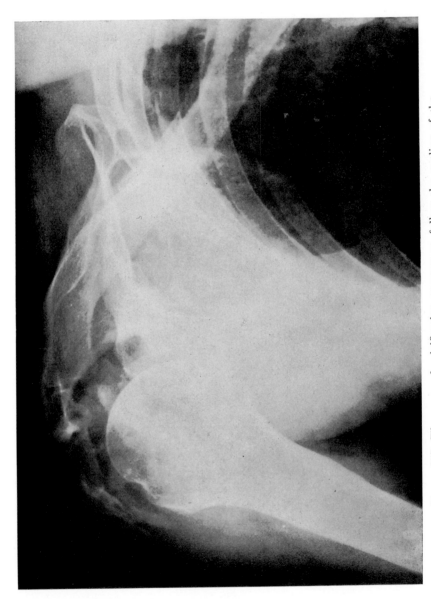

Figure 257. The mass of calcification appears to follow the outline of the deltoid muscle.

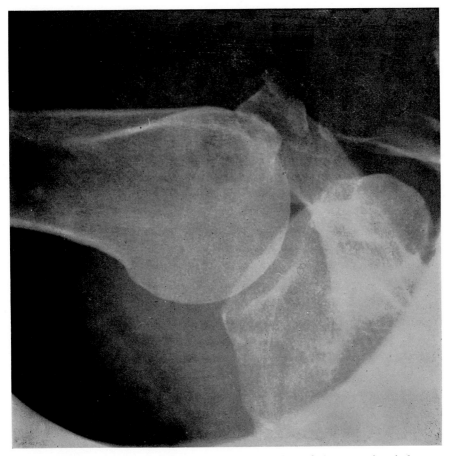

Figure 258. Fracture of the anterior-lateral portion of the acromion is best demonstrated with the arm in some abduction.

one of his feet in the trailer and fell on the street, landing on his right shoulder. He was seen at a compensation clinic the same day. The shoulder was X-rayed and he was told that he had chipped a bone in the shoulder. He had been receiving physical therapy to the shoulder without any relief. He stated that he could not raise his arm above his head and the pain kept him awake at night. Upon clinical examination active abduction was 160 degrees in a slight forward plane. Passive abduction was 120 degrees. Some grating was felt under the acromion when his arm was abducted passively. X-rays were taken and a fracture of the anterior-lateral portion of the acromion was revealed on the anterior-posterior view with the arm in some abduction (Fig. 258).

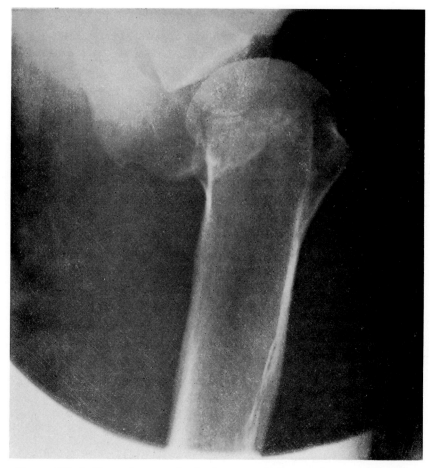

Figure 259. Axillary view reveals the fracture of the anterior portion of the acromion with no evidence of union after seven weeks.

The fracture was also seen on the axillary view (Fig. 259). Since a rupture was also suspected an arthrogram was done and it revealed dye in the subdeltoid bursa (Fig. 260) confirming the clinical findings. At operation, performed a week later, the supraspinatus and infraspinatus tendons were pulled off completely from the greater tuberosity. They were replaced on the tuberosity by making four drill holes in the anatomical neck just medial to the tuberosity. The sutures were placed through these holes and tied below the greater tuberosity. The un-united bone fragment was removed and discarded.

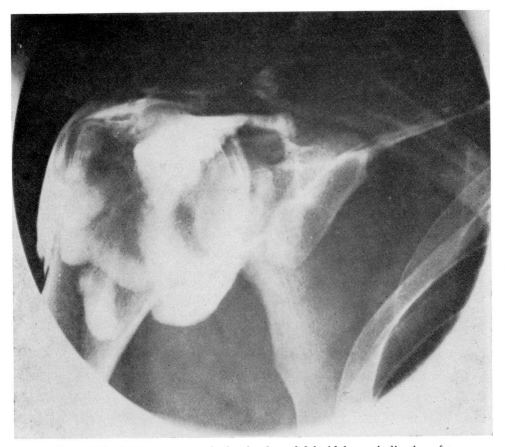

Figure 260. Arthrogram reveals dye in the subdeltoid bursa indicative of a rupture of the rotator cuff.

It is quite evident that a rupture of the rotator cuff must be ruled out in any injury to the acromion, the greater tuberosity or head of the humerus, particularly if a patient continues to have pain, especially at night.

BIBLIOGRAPHY

Axen, P.: Ueber den Wert der Arthrographie des Schultergelenkes. *Acta Radiol, 22:*268–276, 1941.

Bankart, A. S. Blundell: Recurrent or habitual dislocation of the shoulder joint. *Brit Med J, 2:*1132, 1923.

Bankart, A. S. Blundell: The pathology and treatment of recurrent dislocation of the shoulder joint. *Brit J Surg 26:*23, 1938.

Bateman, James E.: *The Shoulder and Neck.* Philadelphia, Saunders, 1972.

Codman, E. A.: *The Shoulder.* Boston, Privately Printed, 1934.

Frostad, H.: Arthrographische untersuchungen des Schultergelenkes, mit spezieller Rücksicht auf die Rupture der sehnen Desselben. *Acta Radiol, 23:*336–353, 1942.

Gasser, G.: Cited by E. Kuster in Ueber Bursitis subacromialis (Periarthritis humero-scapularis). *Arch f Klin Chir, 67:*1013–1021, 1902.

Hill, H. A., and Sachs, M. D.: The grooved defect of the humeral head. A frequently unrecognized complication of dislocations of the shoulder joint. *Radiology, 35:*690–70, 1940.

Kerwein, G. A., Roseberg, Bertil, and Sneed, W. R.: Arthrographic studies of the shoulder joint. *J Bone Joint Surg, 39-A:*1267–1279, December, 1957.

Killoran, Paul J., Marcove, Ralph, and Frieberger, Robert H.: Shoulder arthrography. *American Journal of Roentgenology, 103:* No. 3:658, July, 1968.

Leslie, J. T. and Ryan, T. S.: The anterior axillary incision to approach the shoulder joint. *J Bone Joint Surg, 44A:*1193, 1962.

Lindblom, Knut: Arthrography and roentgenography in ruptures of the tendons of the shoulder joint. *Acta Radiol, 20:*548–562, 1939.

Lindblom, Knut: On pathogenesis of ruptures of the tendon aponeurosis of the shoulder joint. *Acta Radiol, 20:*563–577, 1939.

Lindblom, Knut, and Palmer, Ivar: Ruptures of the tendon aponeurosis of the shoulder joint—The so-called supraspinatus ruptures. *Acta Chir Scandivanica, 82:*133–142, 1939.

Lucas, Donald B.: Biomechanics of the shoulder joint. *Arch Surgery, 107:*425–432, September, 1973.

Moseley, H. F.: *Shoulder Lesions,* 2nd ed. New York, Hoeber, 1953.

Moseley, H. F.: *Recurrent Dislocation of the Shoulder.* Montreal, McGill University Press, 1961.

Moseley, H. F., and Övergaard, M. L.: *Hermodsson's Roentgenological Studies of Traumatic and Recurrent Anterior and Inferior Dislocations of the Shoulder Joint.* Montreal, McGill University Press, 1963.

McLaughlin, Harrison L.: Muscular and tendinous defects at the shoulder and their repair. *Lectures on Reconstruction Surgery,* 343–358, Ann Arbor, Edwards, 1944.

McLaughlin, Harrison L.: Lesions of the musculotendinous cuff of the shoulder, *J Bone Joint Surg, 27:*31, 1944.

Nakaseko, L.: A study of heterotopic ossification, *J Japanese Orthop Assn., 41:*29–44, 1967.

Neviaser, Julius S.: Adhesive capsulitis of the shoulder. A study of the pathological findings in periarthritis of the shoulder. *J Bone Joint Surg, 27:*211–222, April, 1945.

———: An operation for old dislocation of the shoulder. *J Bone Joint Surg, 30-A:*997–1000, October, 1948.

———: Adhesive capsulitis of the shoulder. *Instructional Course Lectures, The American Academy of Orthopaedic Surgeons, 6:*281–191. Ann Arbor, Edwards, 1949.

———: Ruptures of the rotator cuff. *Clinical Orthopaedics, 3:*92–98, Philadelphia, Lippincott, 1953.

———: Injuries in and about the shoulder joint. *Instructional Course Lectures, The American Academy of Orthopaedic Surgeons, 13:*187–216. Ann Arbor, Edwards, 1956.

———: Complicated fractures and dislocations about the shoulder joint. *J Bone Joint Surg, 44-A:*984–998, July, 1962.

———: Adhesive capsulitis of the shoulder. *Medical Times, 90:*783–807, August, 1962.

———: Arthrography of the shoulder joint. Study of the findings in adhesive capsulitis of the shoulder. *J Bone Joint Surg, 44-A:*1321–1330, 1359, October, 1962.

———: Posterior dislocation of the shoulder. Diagnosis and treatment. *Surgical Clinics of N Am, 43:*1623–1630, December, 1963.

———: The treatment of old unreduced dislocations of the shoulder. *Surgical Clinics of N Am, 43:*1671–1678, December, 1963.

———: Musculoskeletal disorders of the shoulder region causing cervicobrachial pain. Differential diagnosis and treatment. *Surgical Clinics of N Am, 43:*1703–1714, December, 1963.

———: Ruptures of the rotator cuff of the shoulder. New Concepts in the diagnosis and operative treatment of chronic ruptures, *Arch Surg, 102:*483–485, May, 1971.

———: Surgical approaches to the shoulder. *Clinical Orthopaedics, 91:*34–40, March–April, 1973.

Oberholzer, J.: Die Arthropneumoradiographie bei habitueller Schulterluxation. *Röntgenpraxis, 5:*589–590, 1933.

Oberholzer, J.: Die Arthro-pneumoradiographie. *Beitr z Klin Chir, 158:*113–156, 1933.

Oberholzer, J.: L'Arthro-pneumoradiographie (méthode de Bircher). *J Radiol et Eléctrol, 20:*15–23, 1936.

Oberholzer, J.: I Methode di contrasto articolari in radiografia. *Chir Organi Movimento, 22:363–372,* 1936–37.

Osmond-Clarke, H.: Habitual dislocation of the shoulder. The Putti-Platt operation. *J Bone Joint Surg, 30-B:19,* 1948.

Pettersson, Gustaf: Rupture of the tendon aponeurosis of the shoulder joint in antero-inferior dislocation. *Acta Chir Scandinivanica, Supplementum, 87,* 1972.

Watson-Jones, Reginald: *Fractures and Joint Injuries,* 4th ed. Baltimore, Williams and Wilkins, 1952, Volume 1, p. 60.

INDEX